Biological Nurturing

Instinctual Breastfeeding

For Jacques

Biological Nurturing

Instinctual Breastfeeding

Suzanne Colson, RM, PhD

2nd Revised and Updated Edition

pinter & martin

DISCLAIMER

The information contained in this publication is advisory only and is not intended to replace sound clinical judgment or individualised patient care. The author disclaims all warranties, whether expressed or implied, including any warranty as the quality, accuracy, safety, or suitability of this information for any particular purpose.

Biological Nurturing: Instinctual Breastfeeding

First published in the US by Hale Publishing 2010

This second UK edition published by Pinter & Martin Ltd 2019
US edition available from Praeclarus Press, LLC

©2019 Suzanne Colson

ISBN 978-1-78066-455-2

Also available as an ebook

British Library Cataloguing-in-Publication Data
A catalogue record for this book is available from the British Library.

Developmental Editing: Kathleen Kendall-Tackett
Additional edit: Sarah Dronfield
Copyediting: Chris Tackett
Based on a layout & design by Nelly Murariu
Index: Helen Bilton

Printed and bound in the EU by Hussar

Pinter & Martin Ltd
6 Effra Parade
London SW2 1PS

pinterandmartin.com

Picture credits:
Fig. 1, 9, 10, 11, 12, 15, 16, 18, 19, 20, 31, 36, 37, 38, 39, 40 © Suzanne Colson
Fig. 5, 27 Fotalia
Fig. 7 first 4 photos © Suzanne Colson, photos 5 and 6 Fotalia, photo 7 © Suzanne Colson
Fig. 8 © Suzanne Colson, except photo 2 Fotalia
Fig. 14 © Suzanne Colson, except photo 5 © Trix Simmons
Fig. 17 line drawings © Francoise Railhet
Fig. 21 top photo © Colson, Frantz & Makelin, bottom photo © Marion Jones
Fig. 22, 25 line drawings © Joelle Dufur
Fig. 23 photos top left and bottom © Suzanne Colson photo top right © Paul Landon
Fig. 24 line drawings © Vicki McGuigan
Fig. 26 line drawing © Sue Carter
Fig. 28 photo © Emma Bader-Devron
Fig. 29 photo on left © Joelle Dufur, middle photo Fotalia, photo on right Dreamstime
Fig. 30 line drawing © Ken Kendell Tackett, photo on right © Suzanne Colson
Fig. 32 © Jack Stern
Fig. 33 First three photos © Fotalia bottom photo on the right © Dreamstime
Fig. 34 photos © Dreamstime
Fig. 35 photo © Johan Hoek

CONTENTS

Acknowledgements   *ix*

Foreword by Kerstin Uvnäs Moberg   *xi*

Foreword by Frédéric Roussel   *xvi*

Preface to the Second Edition   *1*

1: What is Biological Nurturing?   **4**

Practising Biological Nurturing   6

2: Why Do We Need a New Breastfeeding Approach?   **9**

Learning to Breastfeed: Nature or Nurture?   9

The Need for a Different Discourse   15

Shifting the Paradigm   17

3: The Roots of Biological Nurturing   **18**

Personal and Clinical Experience   18

Feeding Records   19

Inspiration from a Landmark Video   20

Beyond the First Hours   21

A Mother/Baby Suckling Diary   22

Overcoming Some Medical Hiccups   23

4: The Biological Nurturing Continuum   **25**

Continuity in Baby Positions   26

Continuity in Baby Reflexes   29

Continuity in Neonatal Behavioural State   29

Continuity for Mothers   31

Continuity of Maternal Hormonal State   31

Biological Nurturing: Keeping Mothers and Babies Together   32

5: Keep the Baby at the Right Address   **33**

Research Case Study   34

Proximity Matters   35

What is Rooming-In?   35

Limitations of Skin-to-Skin Contact   37

Study Review   37

Widström and Colleagues' Interpretations   38

Biological Nurturing Interpretations   38

Is Skin-to-Skin Contact a Habitat?   38
The Right Breastfeeding Address   38
How Long Does It Normally Take a Baby to Find
    the Breast and Latch?   43
Does This Mean That Mothers Shouldn't Practise
    Skin-to-Skin Contact?   48

6 **Transitions: Coping with Discontinuity**   **49**
The First 24 Hours   51
What is Responsive Breastfeeding?   51
Should Mothers Hand Express Even If They Do Not
    Have Any Problems?   52
What Does the Research Say?   53
Active Suckling Matters!   54
The Second 24 Hours   56
What is Discontinuity?   56
Discontinuous Perspectives: The First Hour Following Birth   57
What About the Preterm Baby?   59
When Do Mothers Get Their Milk?   59
How to Know That Baby Is Getting Enough   61
Does That Mean That We Should Never Weigh Babies?   62
The Quest for the Correct Latch   62
The Myth of "Being Settled After A Feed"   62

7 **Exploratory and Descriptive Research**   **65**
The Background Studies of Biological Nurturing   65
An Exploratory Pilot Study   65
Temporal Findings   66
The First 24 Hours   67
The PhD Study of Biological Nurturing   68
Selecting a Research Design   69
What About Skin-To-Skin Contact?   71
Versatility of Early Mother–Baby Contact   74
Understanding Cause and Effect   74
Future Research   74

8 **Biological Nurturing: The Active Ingredients and Mechanisms**   **76**
The Mechanisms of Biological Nurturing   80

9 **Primitive Neonatal Reflexes**   **84**
Schools of Thought on Neurological Assessment   85
The Impact of Neonatal Position   86

What Do PNRs Have to Do with Breastfeeding? 86
Primitive Neonatal Reflexes: Number and Classification 87
The Role Played by PNRs: Unexpected Findings 88
Latch Failure 89
How Does Position Affect the Role of the Reflexes? 91
Dorsal Feeding 91
Frontal Feeding 91
Reflex Activity or Hunger and Interest? 98
The Role of Hunger in Frontal Feeding 98

10 Mother's Breastfeeding Postures 101
Breastfeeding Postures: Research Definitions 102
The Role of the Bony Pelvis 102
The Bony Pelvis 102
Pelvic Sitting Support 104
Postures and Breastfeeding Duration: Research Results 105
Does This Mean That Mothers Should Never Initiate
Breastfeeding in Upright Postures? 108
Maternal Comfort Mechanisms 111
Psychological Comfort: Protecting the Frontal
Region of the Body 112

11 Baby's Breastfeeding Positions 115
What is Lie? 115
What is Neonatal Attitude? 119
What is a Good Fit? 212

12 Lessons from Other Mammals 125

13 Going with Gravity 132
How Can the Milk Flow Up? 133
Parallel Angles on Birth and Breastfeeding 133

14 Neonatal Behavioural State 135
Foetal Life 136
Neonatal Life 136
Doctoral Research: State Definitions and Results 136
Traditional Advice 137
Behavioural State Breastfeeding Mechanisms 139
What Are Feeding Cues? 139
If a Baby's Not Cueing for a Feed, Why Put Him to Breast? 140

Does All This Mean That Mothers Should Sleep with Their Babies? 144
Implications for Practice 145

15 Maternal Hormonal State 147
The Role of Oxytocin 149
Developing Theory 151
Maternal Hormonal Complexion: A Theory 153

16 Instinctual Breastfeeding 155

17 Biological Nurturing: A Mother-Centred Approach 161

Glossary 164
References 171
Appendix: Biological Nurturing Research 185
About the Author 185
Index 186

ACKNOWLEDGEMENTS

I am particularly grateful to the forty breastfeeding mothers who participated in my doctoral research. Thank you so much for sharing your biological nurturing experiences and giving me permission to use your photos and video clips. You have been my teachers. I am also indebted to the many mothers, midwives, doctors, pharmacists, nurses, health visitors and lactation consultants who have written me with insightful comments; some of their testimonials are included throughout the book. I am especially pleased that many newly certified biological nurturing breastfeeding companions (BNCs) have graciously accepted to let me use some of their BN definitions.

I owe a great debt of thanks to Kathy Kendall-Tackett whose editorial skills and guidance transformed an academic doctoral thesis into an easy-to-read book that summarises crucial research findings suggesting that both mothers and babies have an innate capacity to breastfeed. Kathy is a precious friend.

I wish to thank my British publishers, Pinter & Martin, who have kindly waited so patiently for me to finish the revised manuscript. Your constant support and faith has spurred me to have the courage to release new interpretations.

I am indebted to Julia Frimaudeau, a newly certified BNC, who agreed to show us how BN works for her and her newborn baby in the cover photo taken by Paul Landon, a specialist in reflex integration. Paul and his lovely partner, Ludivine Baubry, are unusual; they have been my teachers in navel radiation and the consequences… including developmental delays… associated with not releasing primitive reflexes within the feeding context.

In addition, I remain grateful to Suzanne Carter for the original line drawings and to Vicki McGuigan, a midwife in Nottingham, who has beautifully illustrated the concept of transverse lie.

Last, but certainly not least, I owe a great debt of gratitude to my family. My husband, Jacques, supported me throughout the 1970s and 1980s, where it was nonstop breastfeeding for our three babies. Without this wonderful man, I am not quite sure how I would have made it in life. Jacques was a business consultant and a computer wizard; he helped transform research spreadsheets into easy to understand text, tables, and figures. Our first born, Bertrand, musician, scientist, and statistician, helped clarify the role gravitational forces play; Jean-Christophe, a sociologist, critically appraised each chapter of the book. However, I am particularly indebted to my daughter, Joelle who, at the time of publication, is a third year NHS student nurse. Having followed in my footsteps as a breastfeeding mother of three babies and then a health professional, she has offered precious insight and quality editorial guidance. She also produced the lovely line drawings illustrating foetal and neonatal lie and attitude. Joelle continues to be an inspiring mothering model.

FOREWORD

Kerstin Uvnäs Moberg

Suzanne Colson has written a unique and refreshing book about breastfeeding founded on biology and breastfeeding as a female instinctual ability. She questions present ideas and practices. She shows that women still have the competence to breastfeed, like the first women of the human race and their mammalian sisters, provided they trust their competence and received correct information.

Breastfeeding Is a Natural Inborn Competence

Once upon a time, the ability of women to give birth to children and to breastfeed them was not questioned. Birth and breastfeeding were considered inborn and natural female abilities. Women trusted their competence and rarely experienced any difficulties.

When birth was moved from the mothers' home to hospitals, instinctual behaviours were blocked or extinguished, and innate behaviours were not activated because they were in a completely unnatural environment. Suddenly, women began having problems with birth and breastfeeding. They lost trust in their competence and became convinced that they needed outside help. To cope with these problems, medicalised birth and formula feeding were introduced. Today most women receive some type of medical interventions during birth. In some countries, caesarean section rates are almost 90%, and breastfeeding rates are low despite the large number of scientific studies showing that breastfeeding is better than formula feeding. It promotes health in both infants and mothers not only in developing countries but also in the Western world. There are both short and long term effects.

Reclaiming Women's Natural Capacity to Birth and Breastfeed

A growing group of international researchers, many of whom are female, share the mission of reclaiming the maternal natural competencies. Their goal is to show that women themselves know how to give birth and breastfeed if certain basic requirements are fulfilled. These women work in the health care system often as doctors, nurses, or midwives and are often scientifically trained. By observing the mothers and their babies during birth and breastfeeding, they have demonstrated how hospital environments, medical interventions during birth, and recommendations and practices regarding breastfeeding negatively impact the natural processes of birth and breastfeeding. They propose new practices and recommendations, which are more in line with natural processes, to promote natural birth and breastfeeding. Suzanne Colson is a pioneer and one of the most important persons in this group of researchers.

Biological Nurturing

Suzanne Colson is a brilliant observer, and she has seen how current breastfeeding regimens make it very difficult for women to breastfeed. Professionals' recommendations, both outside and inside hospitals, actually act against biology and the laws of nature and therefore counteract spontaneous breastfeeding. This is why she has created a new manual for breastfeeding that she calls *biological nurturing*. She describes many present routines in detail and explains, based on own observations and scientific data, why they should be avoided. Instead, she advocates several new practices, which are more in tune with natural, spontaneous breastfeeding.

One important aspect of successful breastfeeding is, of course, the mother's feelings of trust and competence. Since the current practices in many ways act against successful breastfeeding, women of today have learned that women can't breastfeed without technical support. Suzanne Colson stresses that professionals need to restore the mothers' self-confidence and trust in themselves as inborn competent breastfeeders, i.e., that breastfeeding is a natural process and that every mother can do it. In this way, professionals should not specifically tell mothers how to breastfeed. Instead, they should make mothers feel comfortable and relaxed, which will bring forward their natural capabilities.

To be fully expressed, like all instinctual behaviours, breastfeeding, or as Suzanne Colson calls it *biological nurturing*, women should be relaxed and not stressed in any way. Maternal posture during breastfeeding should be semi-recumbent. If the mothers are leaning back rather than sitting straight and upright or lying down flat on their backs, which is recommended in many places, relaxation is promoted and thereby, breastfeeding. This recommendation makes sense as this posture actively decreases stress levels and promotes feelings of relaxation.

She also argues that the babies should lie on the mother's breast during breastfeeding. In this way, the baby relaxes and sleeps, ready to latch without too much effort from the mother's part to keep him in place.

Another important observation Suzanne Colson made, which is in line with a positive effect of relaxed states, is that the babies eat well even if they are almost sleeping, which is also against most present knowledge and recommendations. This, however, also makes sense from a basic physiological perspective, since most natural and instinctual behaviours are inhibited not only by stress but also by wakefulness and active concentration. So the more relaxed both mothers and babies are, the better the breastfeeding process will work for both of them.

Who Is Active, Baby or Mother?

There is an interesting controversy in the scientific literature regarding the role of the mother and the infant during breastfeeding. For some, the newborn is the active individual in the breastfeeding situation with the mothers being suppliers of milk in response to the infant's suckling and, in a way, passive observers of the baby's activity. According to these individuals, babies know everything and should govern the entire process and then breastfeeding will work well. Others highlight the role of mothers and see them as active breastfeeders. Suzanne Colson belongs to this second group. She points out that the mother is the more active of the two during breastfeeding, and that they help the babies latch and provide them with milk, warmth, care, and protection, in sync with the baby's demands and reactions. This is an important statement because it is empowering to women to know that they actively breastfeed their babies rather than being reduced to passive observers.

Criticism of Skin-To-Skin Contact

Skin-to-skin contact immediately after birth has become a common practice as a way of increasing the interaction and bonding between mothers and their newborns. This is possibly a modern variant of what was a spontaneous period of closeness chest-to-chest between our ancestral mothers and their newborns as they picked them up to feed and protect them after birth. Suzanne Colson raises objections to some of the ways skin-to-skin contact is implemented. She is critical of the way the newborns are placed on the mother's chest and of the fact that the mothers are lying flat on their backs. Furthermore, she points out that this procedure may make some women feel embarrassed and stressed because they have to be naked and that this may even occur in an unfamiliar place and perhaps with a lot of strangers around. Of course, the presence of unknown persons could be perceived as extremely unpleasant under such circumstances. However, it is important to note that if skin-to-skin contact is performed in a gentle way it should, i.e., in a private and relaxed setting, it is one of the most efficient tools that nature offers to stimulate the interaction between mother and baby and to decrease their stress levels in both the short and long term.

Differences Between Countries

Suzanne Colson performed most of her observational research studies in England, and therefore she bases her criticism of the current system on routines and recommendations of that prevail there. Breastfeeding practices vary between countries, even between European countries, so some of the concerns she raises are not applicable to all countries. But basically, she is correct. Practices that counteract breastfeeding should be abandoned wherever they are used and substituted by new and more optimal recommendations based on the women's natural competence.

Link to Oxytocin

Suzanne Colson often refers to oxytocin, when describing the practices involved in *biological nurturing*. She claims that her recommendations are consistent with "a pulsatile pattern of oxytocin." Oxytocin is a hormone released in response to suckling to stimulate milk ejection during breastfeeding. Oxytocin released from nerves in the brain also plays an important role during breastfeeding. It promotes milk production, decreases levels of anxiety and stress, and increases the mother's interaction with, and bonding to, the baby.

Unfortunately, oxytocin is not always released as it should in modern women, and then the positive effects of oxytocin on milk ejection, milk production, stress levels, and mother's interaction with the baby fail to appear. This is because the oxytocin system was developed hundreds of thousands of years ago, when humans lived under very different circumstances (i.e., as hunters and gatherers). Of course, the biological systems helping mothers with birth and breastfeeding were adapted to the prevailing environment at that time. Certain prerequisites have to be fulfilled for breastfeeding to trigger a maximal release of oxytocin. For example, oxytocin is not released if mothers are stressed or have just concentrated on a mental problem. They need to be relaxed. Furthermore, oxytocin is not released around unknown people and in unfamiliar environments as mothers may unconsciously interpret them as threats, blocking oxytocin release. Therefore, the mother should be in a familiar environment and surrounded by family and close friends when giving birth or breastfeeding.

Suzanne Colson's recommendations within the context of *biological nurturing* make perfect sense also from an oxytocin perspective. Oxytocin simply isn't released if the mother doesn't feel safe, is anxious or stressed, or lacks self-confidence. The breastfeeding practices Suzanne Colson wants to eliminate are those that inhibit the release of oxytocin. By supporting the mother's trust in her competence and her feelings of safety, and by reducing stress and promoting relaxation, oxytocin release is facilitated, and thereby milk ejection, and the other positive physiological and mental effects listed above will be strengthened. In this way, Suzanne Colson's view on breastfeeding and her practical recommendations make deep sense from a physiological point of view. She is opening up for the natural and spontaneous release and effects of oxytocin.

To me, it was fascinating to read Suzanne Colson's book, as the observations and the conclusions she has made, and the recommendations she has put forward fit so well with what is known about oxytocin. The fact that the data obtained from observational studies reflect the present knowledge of the rules for the release and effects of oxytocin strongly supports Suzanne Colson's view on breastfeeding presented in biological nurturing.

Kerstin Uvnäs Moberg, MD, PhD
November 30, 2018

FOREWORD

Frédéric Roussel

I am a practising pharmacist. My wife breastfed our three babies in the 1980s. I accompanied her as best I could… and she, me. We eased into parenting together and this reciprocal journey brimming with mutual discovery, confidence and competence promised a radiant future.

The births of my three children are the best memories of my life, a flashback of happiness that can still make me cry with joy even today. The joy, the pride and the emotion expressed by "ma chérie" while she breastfed our daughter during those two years still resonates in the deepest part of my heart.

In the 1980s, I thought that breastfeeding was a normal, rational choice on many levels: conferring health benefits to babies as well as physiological, anthropological, human, and psychological advantages. I was so naïve; I didn't realise that all of those tins I sold of non-human artificial formula were, in fact, shortening and even aborting the breastfeeding experience.

My wife got me interested in the new breast pumps designed at the turn of the century. From the moment I purchased our first breast pump, an unfurling milky wave buzzed with excitement in my pharmacy. Each day, my team and I spent a great deal of time supporting breastfeeding mothers. I missed seeing mothers when they didn't stop in; normal pharmaceutical life became monotonous. Their visits were a wake-up call yet individual and collective awareness sometimes takes a long time. Little by little I realised how much we didn't know. It was the mothers who knew. But un-learning is the most difficult part. We had to free ourselves from that everlasting cultural paraphernalia that accompanies a bottle feeding culture, things like dummies and bottle teats.

We needed further education and at first training came through luck and then with La Leche League, when an agricultural engineer taught us about Dr. Suzanne Colson's new approach: biological nurturing laid-back breastfeeding. It was an immediate quantum leap; I found my calling: accompanying those courageous mothers who were struggling with breastfeeding.

In 2017, I had the great pleasure of meeting Suzanne Colson, the midwifery doctor in human lactation who leads a most comprehensive breastfeeding workshop emphasising mother-knowledge. The ingredients have always been right there at our fingertips: cupfuls of mothers' innate breastfeeding behaviours, mixed with inborn baby reflexes, and topped with a complicit and tender partnership. Promoting BN marks the final step of a process, the start of which goes back more than 30 years as a practising pharmacist.

Thank you, Dr. Suzanne Colson, for believing that one day pharmacies across the world will respond to mothers' basic needs for accompaniment rather than teaching. Mothers give so much of themselves: their tenderness, their breasts, their milk, their love. We must encourage pharmacists to make time for breastfeeding mothers without prejudice. Like all health professionals, pharmacists have an urgent need for continuous professional development in breastfeeding, free from all competing interests and/or sponsorship.

In the current context, we must relinquish power so that parents reclaim breastfeeding, a SMART objective: specific, measurable, achievable, realistic, and timed.

Frédéric Roussel
Docteur en Pharmacie
Breastfeeding-Friendly Pharmacy, Courbevoie, France

Preface to the Second Edition

This book summarises award-winning doctoral research published in 2008 and introduces biological nurturing (BN), a new approach to breastfeeding. When I wrote the first edition in 2010, I called BN "new" for several reasons. First, midwives and others supporting breastfeeding were consistently taught that human mothers, unlike other mammals, lack breastfeeding instincts. Traditionally, experts have argued that we learn breastfeeding techniques through mimicry and because, as children, we rarely see other mothers breastfeeding their babies, we're hopelessly deficient. Therefore, the role of the health professional is to teach mothers how to breastfeed. Concurrently, experts have always suggested that, unlike other mammals, the human neonate is an obligate dorsal or back-feeder, where pressure is required along the baby's back to keep him in place. This appears to make sense as *Homo sapiens* is the only bipedal, upright primate. BN theory suggests that the human drive to verticality has tacitly influenced maternal breastfeeding positions. From Egyptian times, mothers have been depicted either sitting bolt upright or side-lying to breastfeed. Both positions exert substantial back pressure on the baby.

A second group of reasons leading to a new approach was the recognition of breastfeeding benefits in the 1980s. From a public health perspective, experts introduced breastfeeding management, tightening procedures to avoid conflicting advice, aiming to educate, promote, and support the biological choice. Today, midwifery textbooks in Britain continue to standardise breastfeeding techniques within a "one size fits all" system of latching instructions; the quest for the "correct latch" remains the Holy Grail of breastfeeding.

Having breastfed my babies in the 1970s, before I became a midwife, I never experienced step-by-step procedures; I never knew about the "correct latch" but, like everyone else, I always suggested that mothers use the traditional postures. My doctoral research findings came as a great shock, suggesting that the human neonate, a quadruped at birth, is a ventral or tummy feeder like some of his mammalian cousins.

I studied 40 mother–baby breastfeeding pairs and all were breastfeeding at six postnatal weeks (85% exclusively), yet compelling video data showed mothers and babies breaking all the rules. Human mothers and babies are versatile – able to breastfeed in a variety of positions – and the video clips illustrated that the positions traditionally taught to mothers often (not always) created some of the very problems that they set out to prevent. The data clearly illustrated that the biological nurturing, semi-reclined maternal postures optimised the release of some 20 baby reflexes, enhancing latch and aiding milk transfer.

My research not only reconfigured 17 primitive neonatal reflexes in the feeding context, but the videotaped evidence was also striking, showing how, in BN positions, many mothers acted intuitively; they were often hands-free, enabling them to actively participate. Laid-back breastfeeding was born!

It was an astonishing breakthrough; the BN research findings suggested that the mother's position was central to breastfeeding success. Yet up until 2008, mothers pictured in the mainstream breastfeeding literature were rarely "laid-back." Indeed, when any photo or line drawing showed a mother initiating breastfeeding in a semi-reclined position, there was often a large X placed across it, suggesting that position was wrong.

Today all the Xs are gone from the breastfeeding books but few midwives or professional breastfeeding supporters realise that biological nurturing is much more than a "new" position you're supposed to teach mothers. In particular, BN optimises the baby's position and behavioural state by keeping him at the right address. However, the right address is not placed high on the mother's chest under her chin, or low on her abdomen, positions frequently seen in current mainstream literature. Unsurprisingly, the right address is on the mother's breast. When the baby is on mum's breast, he's either actively feeding or sleeping cheek to breast. Keeping sleeping babies at the right address is good for them. For example, it helps to maintain continuity of womb-feeding frequency as the mammary gland takes over from the placenta. It's also good for mothers, helping them ease into motherhood.

But there's more. Because biological nurturing prioritises maternal comfort, it optimises relaxed, unrestricted baby gazing and eye-to-eye contact at just the right distance. It's well known that these two behaviours promote high oxytocin pulsatility, releasing feelings of maternal love and the spontaneity and reciprocity associated with instinctual breastfeeding.

Laid-back breastfeeding was a catchy term and since the first edition of my book, many health professionals have replaced upright dogma with laid-back dogma, believing that they should actively show all mothers how to breastfeed "naturally" using semi-reclined postures. This is a misunderstanding. Routine teaching is often counterproductive because it stimulates thinking. Planning, thinking, and worrying can suppress spontaneity and overpower instinctual response. Furthermore, many mothers don't want to sit semi-reclined when instructed. Importantly, no research supports the claim that some International Board Certified Lactation Consultants (IBCLCs) have made suggesting that laid-back breastfeeding postures are "natural."

The aim of this second edition is to clarify biological nurturing as a proactive, mother-led, instinctual breastfeeding approach. I have developed further the BN theories, adding five chapters. I have also compared biological nurturing and skin-to-skin contact throughout the book instead of devoting an entire chapter to this.

Mothers are simply amazing and the more I observe them, the more I learn. It's not surprising that when you don't tell mothers what to do, after a brief moment of confusion, they often take the initiative. Taking the lead can be a difficult concept for mothers, having been accustomed to advice, or being shown or told what to do. However, the hit and miss of practising BN is often liberating; mothers soon realise that they're in the driver's seat.

Today, breastfeeding has bad press. Pregnant mothers normally anticipate difficulties and worry that they won't succeed. Antenatal education and mainstream books often plant these seeds of self-doubt, dwelling upon potential breastfeeding problems instead of releasing that spark of joy associated with having a baby. For many mothers it becomes a vicious cycle: the more they read, the more they worry.

We've been terribly unkind suggesting that mothers lack breastfeeding instincts and should, for example, wait to be taught, remain still like lower, small-brained mammals and wait for the baby to do it. It's as though we consider that babies are cleverer than their mothers.

The biological nurturing approach acknowledges maternal competence within a mother–baby relationship, increasing feelings of self-efficacy for both participants. The "mother knows best" wisdom in biological nurturing often initiates a positive chain of relational events that reinforce the lived experience. In other words, breastfeeding can also promote a "virtuous cycle," increasing maternal confidence and enjoyment.

Biological nurturing is quick and easy to do. The watchwords are spontaneity and reciprocity, not advice, teaching, and management. The challenge lies with understanding the releasing mechanisms and their impact. I hope that this book restores your confidence in nature's biological design and in mothers' innate capacity to breastfeed.

CHAPTER 1

What is Biological Nurturing?

Breastfeeding is often promoted as "natural" yet there's widespread scepticism about mothers' instinctive capacity to nourish their babies. This lack of confidence in mothers' innate ability has led health professionals to teach mothers breastfeeding skills and techniques. It is well known that teaching makes people think and usually results in intentional, voluntary behaviour, suppressing spontaneity.

There's a strong argument to suggest that instructing mothers has turned breastfeeding into a catch-22 dilemma. The more you teach a natural process, the more you override instinctual capacity. There's no escape. Or is there?

Biological nurturing (BN) is instinctual breastfeeding and a proactive, mother-centred approach. In BN, maternal comfort is a priority. Mothers relax in semi-reclined positions and that's why in 2008, I introduced the term "laid-back breastfeeding".[1] However, BN is much more than a semi-reclined posture. Biological nurturing is a collective term for mother–baby positions and states that interrelate and interact to release primitive neonatal reflexes and spontaneous maternal breastfeeding behaviours. Figure 1 illustrates the BN components.

Look at Figure 1. Do you see that each component is half mother and half baby? That's because biological nurturing highlights the breastfeeding relationship. Optimising hormonal state for mothers is as important as ensuring she's in a comfortable, laid-back position. All midwives know that high maternal oxytocin during labour usually leads to a spontaneous birth. Likewise, high oxytocin pulsatility releases intuitive breastfeeding. The assessment of the mother's hormonal state is paramount and one way in which BN differs from traditional breastfeeding approaches. Importantly,

Figure 1: Biological Nurturing Components

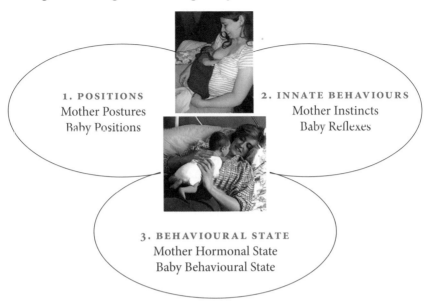

1. POSITIONS
Mother Postures
Baby Positions

2. INNATE BEHAVIOURS
Mother Instincts
Baby Reflexes

3. BEHAVIOURAL STATE
Mother Hormonal State
Baby Behavioural State

hormonal state is often linked to posture, another BN component. A breastfeeding mother sitting upright trying to remember latching instructions reminds us of Rodin's famous sculpture. *The Thinker* sits upright, muscles tensed, leaning forward with furrowed brow. In contrast, the mother practising BN, sits semi-reclined; she often has glazed eyes, a half-smile, a facial blush, and low body tone while gazing at her baby. These latter characteristics are associated with high levels of oxytocin.

The BN research data clearly show that the role of the health professional is to manage the environment, not to teach positioning and attachment. The priority for physiological acts like childbirth and breastfeeding is to promote high maternal oxytocin pulsatility. When you do, it's like magic; even a slight change in maternal posture often unleashes a breastfeeding gene, hidden under layers of cultural warping.

There is an evolutionary argument suggesting that any act that ensures the survival of the species would logically bring rewards. The positional components of biological nurturing reward mothers by reducing the muscle tension and fatigue that many of them experience in upright postures. This in turn increases enjoyment, which may help sustain breastfeeding. People tend to continue doing the things they enjoy.

Gravity plays an important role in every life-sustaining act. Biological nurturing makes use of gravity to help babies latch; this is another gift because research shows that mothers always sacrifice their own comfort for a latch that works.[2] Going with gravity reduces breast fighting, sore nipples, and other problems that have traditionally made mothers stop breastfeeding before they intended.

Practising Biological Nurturing

Biological nurturing is quick and easy to do. There's nothing to remember, no correct latch, no step-by-step instructions for mothers, but there are some general guidelines for health professionals. First, don't try to teach mothers a new, "natural" breastfeeding posture. Instead, encourage mothers to get comfortable. Many mothers don't want to lean back if you suggest that they sit semi-reclined, but no one ever refuses comfort. We explore this stance further in Chapter 12, explaining a human positional paradox.

In biological nurturing, what's important is that the mother's back is supported, touching the back of the chair, sofa, or bed. You'll want to ensure that every part of her body can relax (especially her shoulders, neck, and arms). Observe her: if her muscles remain tense, ask her how she usually watches television. Many mothers are comfortable breastfeeding in those positions. Be aware that no mother should lie flat or almost flat on her back, and that the optimal degree of recline varies from mother to mother. Importantly, the position that works best ensures comfortable baby gazing and/or mother–baby eye-to-eye contact.

Finally, encourage mothers to take the lead. Suggest that they place their sleeping babies on top of their bodies, keeping them there for as often and as long as desired, but at least for an hour; during 60 minutes of sleep, the baby completes at least one, maybe two or even three sleep cycles. In my doctoral study, more than a third of the babies latched on in light or drowsy sleep states. Importantly, all of the breastfeeding mothers ($n=40$) practised BN and all were breastfeeding at six postnatal weeks (85% exclusively).[3] We will explore newborn babies' sleep in depth in Chapter 14.

"Spontaneous, instinctual, intuitive, involuntary, and reciprocal" are the watchwords and once in BN positions, breastfeeding often becomes an innate mother–baby dance, not taught baby-led steps.[4]

Look at video clip 1 below. Do you see how the baby's thighs, calves, and feet tops are in close body contact? They brush up against mum's body, releasing, placing, and stepping. Many health professionals think that skin-to-skin contact releases these reflexes. However, the mechanisms of biological nurturing clearly show that, for the baby, it's a combination effect: constant tummy pressure and movement from body brushing release these inborn reflexes, not nudity. Although many mothers love the feel of full bare-skin contact, some

Video 1: An innate mother-baby breastfeeding dance

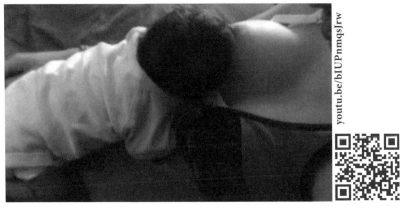

youtu.be/bIUPnmqsJrw

Like their babies, mothers are hardwired to breastfeed, and in Video Clip 1 you can observe a mother who, without any instruction, instinctively places her baby, gently helping him latch when necessary.

do not. Some mothers get hot and perspire. Others are embarrassed or feel uncomfortable at the very thought of being naked even if a blanket covers them. Just as there's not one position for breastfeeding, there's not one dress state. Positions and dress state change depending upon the environment and personal preferences.

That means that you can BN your baby anywhere, anytime – in the privacy of your home or when you're out and about. Mothers should therefore be made aware that breastfeeding positions and dress state are always their individual choice.

Look at Video Clip number 2.

Video 2: Don't wake the baby. Babies, sleeping at the right address, latch on and feed

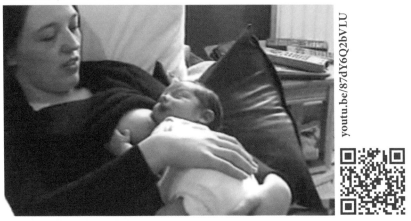

youtu.be/87dY6Q2bVLU

Tummy pressure and body brushing movements are such powerful releasers that this baby latches on even when in light sleep and drowsy states.

People often ask me: "Why would anyone put a sleeping baby to breast?" The simple answer is because babies latch on and feed. Importantly, don't wake the baby! When you want a sleeping newborn to breastfeed, just BN her for an hour or so. The BN mother–baby positions interact in the same way as when baby is awake, resulting in involuntary reflex movements that aid latch. We will explore how ventral pressure works in Chapter 4 and have an in-depth discussion of reflex behaviours in Chapter 9.

But there's more. Importantly, when you BN your sleeping baby, you keep him in the human biological habitat or what I call the right address.[5] In BN, when the baby's sleeping, his cheek usually lies on mum's bare breast but, as stated above, ventral or abdominal nudity is neither necessary for mother nor for baby. Mothers and babies breastfeed beautifully well when both are lightly dressed.

Finally, just sitting in laid-back positions promotes comfortable baby gazing and eye-to-eye contact; both increase oxytocin pulsatility.[6] Throughout this book we will explore how mother–baby positions and states interrelate and interact because these are the variables that unlock instinctual breastfeeding.

CHAPTER 2

Why Do We Need a New Breastfeeding Approach?

Introducing a new approach for an age-old art is a monumental task and many people are both intrigued and confused about biological nurturing. People often ask: "Why do we need a new breastfeeding approach? What's the matter with the old one?"

First and foremost, biological nurturing recognises the mother's instinctual breastfeeding competence, whereas the current paradigm validates the role of the health professional imparting their expert knowledge.[1] Most mothers initiate breastfeeding in hospital and feeding the infant has become a medicalised act with a focus on skills-teaching and management.

Although research in the 1990s finally recognised that human babies are born competent, able to find the breast, self-attach, and feed,[2] unfortunately, human mothers are not credited with the same expertise. Lactation consultants often say that breastfeeding is "natural," yet they teach mothers how to do it. This is confusing; an approach where you teach what's believed to be instinctive is an oxymoron.

Biologically, mothers would normally inherit the genetic capacity to feed the offspring, ensuring the survival of the species. From a biological nurturing perspective, the question to ask is how do human mothers develop these instincts? Is breastfeeding completely innate or is it wholly learned?

Learning to Breastfeed: Nature or Nurture?

This question is at the heart of the discourse around breastfeeding approaches and how best to support mothers. It is also part of a larger discussion that permeates our understanding of child development. *Nature* refers to a person's innate characteristics or dispositions. Those supporting the nature perspective of the origins of behaviour argue that a person's capacity to act instinctively is inborn, not learned.

Simply put, an innate behaviour is an action, a movement you can see, or a sound you can hear, and there are two basic types: reflexes and instincts. In both, the behaviour is involuntary, spontaneous, and/or hardwired, a part of our genetic inheritance, built into the brain before birth.

Innate behaviour is released by internal or external stimuli, or a combination of the two. Desmond Morris, author of fabulous books on people and baby watching, suggests that there are basically two kinds of genetically pre-programmed behaviours: inborn reactions and discovered behaviours or those uncovered through the hit-and-miss of the experience.[3]

Tinbergen and Lorenz, Nobel-prize-winning ethologists, observed animals in their natural environments. They defined five basic endogenous drives that release those inborn or discovered behaviours that ensure the survival of the species.[4,5] These are often termed the five Fs: fleeing, fighting, freezing, feeding, and mating.

In contrast, *nurture* means nourish, develop, bring up (or raise), discipline or educate. Nurturing is learned behaviour and ranges from early feeding choices to opening a bank account for your child. The advocates of the nurture determinant of behaviour consider that the baby is born like a clean slate ready for experiences to write his behavioural capacity. Epidemiological variables, such as ethnicity, age, geographic situation, education, income, social class and other socioeconomic factors, are "nurture." Environmental influences are central to the determination of human achievement.[6] This is the public health perspective.

In the breastfeeding world, the current dominant paradigm leans heavily towards the "nurture" end of the spectrum, highly influenced by a public health approach. "Enable," "consistency of advice," "policy," "guidelines," and "targets" are some public health watchwords.

Public health, informed by epidemiology, is defined as a field of medicine that deals with the physical and mental health of the community. It's a four to five step process, which includes promotion, education, support, and protection, sometimes leading to legislation. Initially, public health doctors focused almost entirely upon sanitation: a clean water supply, waste disposal, and food safety.[7]

In the 18th century, William Cadogan, a physician, recognised food safety as an important public health issue. Infant mortality was rampant and Cadogan medicalised nursing practices, advocating a "return to nature," hardiness, and breastfeeding in an attempt to strengthen infants' resistance against disease.

This led to a science of infant feeding with strict schedules in a backlash against "soft" mothering practices and "feminine errors of judgment." The opening sentence of his essay reveals the origins of a public health, management approach that was to become the dominant mindset.[8]

> *It is with great Pleasure I see at last the Preservation of Children become the Care of Men of Sense. In my opinion, this Business has been too long fatally left to the management of Women, who cannot be supposed to have proper Knowledge to fit them for such a Task, notwithstanding they look upon it to be their own Province.*

Hardyment, an English historian, calls Cadogan's essay the first of the baby care manuals written by the "enlightened male expert." This marked the advent of a man's discourse into the baby care arena, an area which was previously uniquely feminine.[9]

Early in the 20th century Sir Frederick Truby King, another "enlightened physician," firmly anchored the need for medical instruction and management within the mainstream breastfeeding discourse:

> *Just as the whole subject of Mothercraft does not come by instinct to a woman the moment she becomes a mother, but has to be studied, so does breast-feeding require thoughtful study and competent management if it is to be a success.*[10]

Sir Truby King expanded management techniques to include advice suggesting that too much baby holding would spoil babies, driving them to a feckless adulthood. Although he passionately endorsed breastfeeding, he introduced the notion of the "good baby," requiring mothers to establish "good habits" from birth, producing "a perfectly happy and beautiful Truby King baby," writes his adopted daughter in a manual called *Mothercraft*.[11]

The nurturing approach aims to standardise procedures, promoting consistency of advice. However, the biological argument suggests that it's difficult to standardise practices associated with human life sustaining acts. This drive towards standardization can create a real tension between nature and nurture. In the past, that often led to heated debate across disciplines.

Today, experts now agree that both nature and nurture act and interact to influence behaviours and developmental outcomes.[12] However, currently, the genetic or instinctual ways of knowing are not recognised as playing an important part in how mothers develop the capacity to breastfeed. Instead, people attribute the acquisition of breastfeeding behaviours to mimicry and skills-teaching.

Mavis Gunther, a well-known English obstetrician and breastfeeding expert, stated categorically that mothers lack breastfeeding instincts.[13]

> There can be no doubt in the minds of those taking care of modern Western European and American women...that instinct does not inform the mother how to feed her first baby...which is all the more remarkable since labour which is part of the same job is more effectively compulsive.

This paper, published in *The Lancet*, a highly respected peer-reviewed medical journal, may be at the root of modern "nurture" or public health dominance in breastfeeding. However, it should be noted that Gunther did not base her observations on research but rather on her clinical experience. Having read Tinbergen and Lorenz, Gunther was puzzled and sought to clarify the causes of what she considered this "maternal breastfeeding deficiency." She theorised that in primates, including *Homo sapiens*, mimicry takes the place of instinct. She supported her argument by citing, what was at the time, recent news about a chimpanzee born in captivity who gave birth at London Zoo and rejected the baby. If it hadn't been for the kindly zookeepers who fed it, the baby chimp would have died.

Eight years after the publication of Gunther's landmark paper, Karen Pryor, an American marine biologist who wrote one of the first books about breastfeeding for mothers, recounts the incident:

> A chimpanzee reared in the London Zoo had never seen a baby of her own species. She was so horrified at the sudden appearance of her first baby in her nice, safe and hitherto private cage that she leapt backwards with a shriek of terror and could never thereafter be persuaded to have anything to do with her offspring.[14]

Observations like these across the industrialised world led health professionals to embrace Gunther's deterministic explanation for breastfeeding failure. Human mothers, living in a bottle feeding culture, were deprived of the visual experience of breastfeeding as children. Like animals born and raised in captivity, this deprivation during childhood resulted in maternal rejection of the offspring at birth and the inability to breastfeed.

Today, other interpretations are possible. Women having their babies in hospital are closely observed and must comply with hospital policy. Interestingly, they often use prison language, suggesting tacit feelings of captivity, saying, for example: "I didn't know I was allowed to hold my baby" or "tomorrow I will be released" instead of saying they are going home.

Feeling observed in an unfamiliar environment is known to suppress spontaneity, creativity, and innate behaviour. This might explain why women, giving birth in hospital, often look to health professionals for guidance. This likely reduces oxytocin pulsatility. Gunther's conclusion that women need to be taught the skills of breastfeeding set the context for the public health approach to lean almost entirely towards the "nurture" end of the spectrum.

Although BN has become accepted practice in many countries, Gunther's approach continues to guide breastfeeding support in the two British textbooks that shape midwifery education. British midwives learn that two maternal breastfeeding positions are "correct": sitting upright or side-lying. There are no line drawings of mothers and babies breastfeeding in BN positions. In the most recent edition of *Myles Textbook for Midwives*, Midwife Sally Inch[15] writes that mothers should avoid "chairs with a deep backward sloping seat," in other words, comfortable chairs. Inch continues to teach that the upright position enhances the shape of the breast although there is no research to support that statement. Nevertheless, midwives are expected to assess "the angle that mothers' breasts dangle" instead of maternal comfort.

The emphasis is on "correct" techniques for milk transfer, not enjoyment. For example, mothers must hold their babies nipple-to-nose and lead swiftly in with the chin following mouth gape. Inch also states that it may help to swaddle the baby in a small sheet so that his hands are by his sides. In other words, she advocates suppressing the baby's searching reflexes.

Inch's approach illustrates what Burns and her colleagues call the dominant "breastmilk as 'liquid gold' discourse"; 80% of the midwives in their study considered themselves to be the expert clinician, "teacher and supervisor of the woman's use of her breastfeeding equipment".[16]

It's no wonder that I continue to receive testimonials like the one below where I have combined a number of points received from distressed mothers.

◆

TESTIMONIAL

My daughter was placed to my breast shortly after the birth in skin-to-skin contact; she sucked and fed and sucked and fed – it was fabulous. My midwife had heard of your approach. She was relaxed and simply placed her there; I was a bit out of it and my baby did her own thing; I laid back, looked at her, and finally relaxed! I decided there and then that breastfeeding was definitely for me but was very apprehensive, as I had heard so many negative things regarding breastfeeding. Incredibly, none of my friends had been successful for any length of time. I am certain that if my midwife had not been so natural and chilled out about this first feed things would have been very different for me!

When I was moved to the postnatal ward a few hours after the birth, it was horrendous. Midwives standing guard scrutinising every move I made breast-wise, comparing what I did to midwifery textbooks! It was here that I heard that my breasts did not dangle the right way… "nipple to nose" spoken aloud revealed that my nipples were down by my waist. I had read about breastfeeding before having my baby but didn't realise there were procedures almost treated as the law! I hate all that now.

The midwives said that the videos I'd seen on YouTube didn't work. They were just for show. They suggested that I needed to sit upright…I was intimidated and did what they said. Then one of the midwives stood in front of me watching me, saying that I was doing it all wrong and she forced my baby onto the breast. They said I couldn't go home until she was gaining weight and I couldn't manage to do that so I said OK even though I wanted to be out of there. I tried to let her find her way to the nipple and was immediately berated for it!

Please tell other mothers. I would have appreciated simply being told that there are alternative ways to breastfeed! The hospital staff was obsessed with breastfeeding without seeming to offer any practical advice except for the instructions printed in the government leaflets. I have learned now that, as a mother, your instincts CAN be trusted and that your baby is well equipped to feed himself given half a chance. I just needed someone to tell me this at the time!

Thank you so much for introducing BN, which has given me so much reassurance and a lot more confidence about things. I hope I can pass this on to any new mums I come into contact with through my peer supporting role in the future.

◆

Burns and her colleagues found that a majority of midwives consider that mothers lack the knowledge and skill development to breastfeed. Women are therefore encouraged to call the "expert" who will show them how to breastfeed. The "expert" even offers unsolicited help and consistent advice such as:

- Sit upright with feet flat on the floor or lie on your side.
- Be relaxed and comfortable.
- Ensure your breasts are hanging naturally.

Then …

- Use one of three holds.
- Bring baby in close.
- Place the baby nipple to nose.
- Wait for mouth gape.
- Lead in with the chin.
- Ensure baby's chin/mouth or lower lip touches the breast first.
- Align the baby's head and body.
- Ensure the baby's lower lip is turned outward.
- Hear no noise other than swallowing.[17, 18, 19]

The biological nurturing perspective suggests that these instructions take away the joy of breastfeeding. However, they are the breastfeeding basics, a prescriptive discourse that UK midwives are taught to use to support mothers, some of which we see in the testimonial above. It is as though the purpose of breastfeeding, like bottle feeding, is to get milk into a baby. Is it not time to recognise maternal instinctual competence and renew our breastfeeding vocabulary?

The Need for a Different Discourse

Many people ask me: "Why do you have to introduce new terminology? Why can't you just call it breastfeeding?" Again, there are many reasons. Importantly, breastfeeding has bad press as we have just seen in the above testimonial. Many mothers are apprehensive as soon as they become pregnant. They worry about myriad things that their friends have experienced including sore nipples and fear of embarrassment while breastfeeding out and about.

The focus of the words "breastfeeding" and "breastmilk" is BREAST; the equivalent in the animal world would be to call cow's milk "udder milk." This terminology objectifies "the breast" as equal to "the bottle" and subtly bypasses the mother's nurturing role. In other languages, for example, in French, breastfeeding is called mother feeding (*l'allaitement maternel*).

It's hard to believe but in many circles in the industrialised world, breast-feeding in public remains taboo. Many people become angry or upset at the mere thought of a naked breast in the mammary context. BN shifts the emphasis to more discreet nurturing behaviours because in BN most babies are already asleep on the breast. Even though legislation protects breastfeeding in public, it is often frowned upon. For example, waiters in a well-known London restaurant recently covered a mother and her baby from neck to toe in a white tablecloth while she breastfed during dinner.

In stark contrast, the blatantly naked breast continues to be treated as something to be admired and celebrated in a sexual context, in adult magazines or tabloids, for example. In stock photos or mainstream literature, breastfeeding mothers are often depicted naked, establishing a tacit mindset about dress state. These opposing representations of women's breasts confuse the mammary function with more explicit sexual undertones.

Of course mothers can breastfeed discreetly but health professionals are increasingly prescribing X amount of hours of skin-to-skin contact during the first postnatal week.[20] Many mothers think that they must lie down naked in bed to do it. Rules making place and dress state explicit can also infringe upon a mother's power of decision-making. Women can experience embarrassment, or shame, even when they're at home.

For example, I was asked to visit a new mother experiencing latching problems. I found her sitting upright in her bed in bare skin-to-skin contact with her 3 day old baby. Her husband and mother-in-law were in attendance. Both of them, fully dressed, were peering at her, suggesting solutions. When I entered her bedroom, she burst into tears, apologising for her perceived body odour, saying that she was hot and had been in skin-to-skin for hours although baby had not yet latched. This mother's privacy was breached, and she felt embarrassed, confused, and out of control. Once she had showered and dressed, her then-sleeping baby latched on almost immediately during biological nurturing.

Finally, in midwifery textbooks, there are no breastfeeding chapters. Instead, breast and bottle-feeding are grouped together under "Infant Feeding" as though they are equivalent methods.[21, 22] Entwistle has taken a refreshing approach, introducing infant feeding as part of the mother–baby relationship. However, throughout her chapter the traditional breastfeeding beliefs prevail with rhetoric and drawings of mother–baby positions similar to the Inch model.

Breastfeeding is nothing like bottle feeding. That doesn't mean that mothers who choose to bottle feed don't need support, or that they won't establish loving, close relationships with their babies. But here we are talking about midwifery education. Student midwives need to learn how to support both breastfeeding and bottle feeding mothers. For example, bottle feeding is not an innate behaviour; mothers DO need step-by-step instructions to learn how to mix infant formula. Combining the two in one chapter suggests that the support is identical. This prevents student midwives from learning how to prioritise mother knowledge as central to their breastfeeding experiences.

People often say: "Yes, but it's not politically correct to separate the two feeding methods; bottle feeding mothers might feel guilty." Of course, midwives are often mothers who bottle fed their own babies; however, as with any profession, personal feelings and experiences should not cloud professional knowledge and judgement. Also, midwives need to be consistent.

Despite many mothers requesting no-labour caesarean sections, midwives promote normal vaginal birth. The midwifery textbooks do not combine normal vaginal birth and birth by caesarean section in one chapter entitled "Birth." The way mothers are accompanied and birth is managed, and any deviation from the normal is detected, varies according to the mother's individual circumstances.

These arguments suggest that it's inappropriate to have breast and bottle-feeding in one chapter. It is time to emphasise these distinctions so that student midwives learn to promote and support breastfeeding yet validate all mothers in their choices.

Shifting the Paradigm

BN brings "nature to the fore," attempting to restore a balance by shifting the paradigm back to where the "nature" end of the spectrum is once again included.[23] From an evolutionary perspective, it doesn't make sense that mothers would lack breastfeeding instincts. With this in mind, the words "biological nurturing" in themselves suggest that we develop the capacity to breastfeed in a variety of different ways that include both instinctual and learned behaviour. The concept of "biological nurturing" enables us to reappraise our priorities, attempting to highlight maternal nurturing competence. Understanding how the BN components interact compels us to identify some breastfeeding myths, received ideas, and unsupported assumptions passed down by those with a more medicalised, public health approach.

It has been almost 300 years since breastfeeding became a taught medical event. Is it not time for mothers to reclaim their breastfeeding gene and the discourse that places mothers in the limelight? BN is a new, instinctive approach to breastfeeding and may be a precious resource, awakening innate mother knowledge.

CHAPTER 3

The Roots of Biological Nurturing

B iological nurturing has been developed over the past 25 years through personal and clinical experience, and research and practice-development projects. Before looking at the theories of why biological nurturing works, and the research that examines what makes it work, we need to review how BN was first developed. This review is an attempt to clarify the concept further and provide some background information on how this concept evolved.

Personal and Clinical Experience

As the mother of three breastfed infants, and a founder of La Leche League France, I worked as a lactation consultant for three years at Pithiviers State Hospital, a pioneering French birth centre. Highly influenced by what I learned about the connections between birth and breastfeeding during that time, I decided to become a midwife. Upon qualification, I worked for a short time as a caseload midwife and then returned to specialise in infant feeding, supporting both breast and bottle-feeding mothers in hospital and the community.

Although bottle-feeding mothers sometimes have problems, more breast-feeding mothers – up to 20 a day – wanted my help. I relied upon the counselling skills acquired as a La Leche League Leader, together with my midwifery training, to help them.[1] My work with mothers ranged from simple verbal encouragement to hold the baby to more complex situations requiring clinical intervention, such as where mothers had sore, bleeding nipples, mastitis, or medical conditions, like hypertension and caesarean-wound infections. I gained experience across a wide range of different clinical situations. These typically included healthy term, preterm, or small-for-gestational-age neonates, dehydrated and/or failure-to-thrive infants requiring readmission to hospital, and previously sick babies, normalising breastfeeding in preparation for hospital discharge from special care.

Feeding Records

Charting feeds is part of routine postnatal midwifery assessment, and standard forms are provided by most UK hospitals. Although there are small variations, feeds are recorded in a column labelled Type of Feed. Other columns indicate Amount Offered, Amount Taken, Vomit, Urine, and Bowel Output.

Although the charts were used for both breast and bottle-feeding mothers, the information focused exclusively on bottle-feeding. For example, midwives often wrote the commercial trademark of the artificial milk drink* offered for type of feed, and a column for vomit appeared to be included because artificially fed babies often bring up large quantities of the commercial milk drink.

Clinical experience suggested that this column was unnecessary for breastfed babies, as they rarely have milk vomits in the first postnatal days. The amount-offered and amount-taken columns seemed to undermine breastfeeding. Midwives often noted the time at the breast as an indication of the amount taken. The record of the amount ingested was considered important because it could then be compared to pre-calculated milk volumes based upon energy requirements. At the time, this was 60–100 ml/kg/day, which is an assumption driven by a bottle-feeding culture.

As we have seen previously, breastfeeding research demonstrates that these volumes are likely too much, especially in the first 24 hours.[2,3] Furthermore, more recent research suggests that these larger quantities of artificial milk drink may have a negative impact upon the physiological processes involved in metabolic adaptation.[4,5] Nevertheless, these were the volume indicators commonly used to inform all assessments of neonatal well-being.

The charts in themselves seemed to plant seeds of doubt, encouraging supplementation with artificial milk drink even when breastfed babies appeared to be thriving. I was often discouraged by the amount of time

---

* I call all commercial breastmilk substitutes "artificial milk drink" not "baby milk," as it is commonly termed in Britain. Just as a commercial orange juice that is not made with oranges must legally be called orange drink not orange juice, baby milk that is not human should be called artificial milk drink.

wasted crossing out the chart headings and explaining breastfeeding parameters to the mothers. See Figure 2 for a typical British feed chart.

Figure 2: Typical British Feed Chart

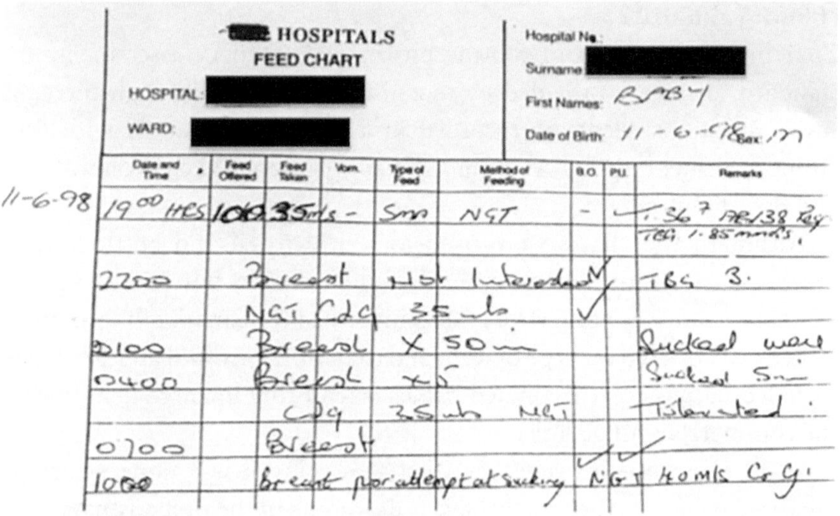

Inspiration from a Landmark Video

Things started to change for me when I first saw Kittie Frantz's video production, *Delivery Self-Attachment*. At the time, I was a midwife/babyfeeding advisor, responsible for two busy postnatal wards in a large London hospital. This six minute video[6] stimulated ideas about new ways to support breastfeeding.

The video displayed clips from an observational study and showed mothers and babies in the first postnatal hour. The aim of the research was to examine the effects of early mother/baby separation at birth upon breastfeeding. Seventy-two mothers self-selected to one of two groups: a *contact group*, where they had at least an hour of uninterrupted skin-to-skin contact with their babies following birth or until the first breastfeed, or a *separation group*, where the neonate had skin-to-skin contact with the mother for about 20 minutes after the birth but was then removed for measuring, bathing, and dressing before being returned to the mother.

Infants in the contact group displayed crawling, stepping, and the rooting reflex, as well as mouthing movements after about 20 minutes. At 50 minutes, most had self-attached and were suckling. Ten infants in the contact group, whose mothers received intramuscular injections of pethidine (Demerol, USA trademark), a narcotic analgesic for pain relief during labour, did not self-attach spontaneously during the first postnatal hour. Most infants in the separation group, when returned to their mothers, had no sense of direction and displayed a poor suckling technique. Righard and Alade concluded that babies should be left undisturbed in skin-to-skin contact with their mothers during the first hour following birth and that narcotic analgesia should be restricted.

These recommendations were challenged, at the time, as the relatively small groups were drawn from a convenience sample, not randomised. Furthermore, the type of pain relief was not deemed relevant at the outset of the study and was therefore poorly controlled, not being held constant across the groups. Breastfeeding definitions were not made explicit and observers of suckling technique were not blinded to the group allocation.[7,8] However, the video clips were appealing and invited discussion during my weekly antenatal education sessions for parents.

Frequent viewings prompted me to think about my practice. Further reflection led to concepts central to the development of BN as an early postnatal intervention. For example, the maternal body appeared to provide some continuity from foetus to neonate, suggesting that it would, perhaps, be an ideal nurturing environment not only for the first hour following birth but also during the establishment of breastfeeding.

In the video, a clip showed the behaviour of a baby who had been separated from his mother. The baby did not appear to have a sense of direction and did not latch. However, he did make some gross rooting movements from side to side. I wondered whether prolonged mother–baby contact in those same close frontal positions could rescue the full reflex.

Beyond the First Hours

Mothers and babies are often separated immediately following birth for a variety of baby-centred reasons, including foetal distress, birth asphyxia, caesarean section, ventouse or forceps deliveries, prematurity, and any other intercurrent situation demanding facial oxygen or full resuscitation. Some mothers also require care necessitating separation or where baby holding is difficult. Other mothers request a meal, a bath or shower, or they feel too exhausted to hold the baby. Viewing and reviewing these video clips led to other theoretical questions:

1. Could prolonged baby holding in close body contact during the first postnatal days help to compensate for such delays in breastfeeding initiation?
2. Would it be possible for reluctant, slow feeders, or those babies recovering from birth in mothers' arms, to self-attach as the babies did in the video and feed well at a later stage?

The early patterns of crawling and mouthing looked like involuntary movement and appeared to be triggered by neonatal positions on the maternal body even when the baby seemed to be asleep. Another question surfaced: could all babies feed in sleep states, as the one in the video appeared to do? This got me thinking and I made immediate changes in my clinical practice.

A Mother/Baby Suckling Diary

First, I adapted the feed charts, changing the terminology to reflect breastfeeding needs. For example, instead of being called a feed chart, it became a mother/baby suckling diary. Mothers, not midwives, kept the diary. Breastfeeding was called suckling because, by definition, suckling is a mother/baby activity and the word in itself was abstract, playing down the need to "fill the baby up" inherent in the "feed" part of breastfeeding.

Physiological and relational grounds were introduced to encourage baby holding, using words like cues and responses borrowed from the Kangaroo Mother Care literature.[9] Maternal cues were explained as those behaviours inviting the baby to feed, for example, brushing the baby's lips with the maternal nipple. Baby cues included sucking on hands or fingers, lip smacking, rooting movements during light sleep and were discussed as early indicators of feeding readiness.

I encouraged mothers to look for these behaviours, recording them and any other details concerning their relationship with their babies. I also told them to pick up their sleeping babies and to hold them at the breast for long periods of time. The diaries revealed that the longer mothers held their babies, the more they fed. Therefore, the diary was expanded to include an enlarged meaning of "demand feed" to include maternal "demand." This encouraged mothers to hold and suckle their babies for as long as they wanted, regardless of the time the baby actively fed.

The routine teaching of positioning and attachment skills during the first day quickly became unnecessary. Instead, based upon previous learnings from La Leche League, together with the growing body of evidence supporting Kangaroo Mother Care, I encouraged mothers to offer unrestricted access to the breast for as long as they wanted, in as much skin-to-skin contact as they wanted. Healthy term babies are born well fed. The key priority just after birth became "enjoyment," not feeding.

Overcoming Some Medical Hiccups

But was it safe to allow mothers to have this much freedom, without the constant charting and management by health professionals? One concern doctors immediately raised was neonatal hypoglycaemia. Hypoglycaemia, defined as low circulating blood sugar concentrations, is often seen as a risk for any baby who does not appear to be ingesting the "correct" weight/ volume amounts discussed above.

At the time, research by Hawdon and her colleagues had been published and their results clearly demonstrated that the healthy term breastfed neonate, unlike his bottlefed cousin, produces ketone bodies when blood sugar concentrations are in the lower ranges of normal. It is well recognised that the human brain is an obligate consumer of glucose. Nevertheless, ketone bodies are now accepted as an alternative source of fuel for the neonatal brain during the first three postnatal days, the time of metabolic adaptation.[10,11,12] Called suckling ketosis, this neonatal capacity to counter-regulate is unique among mammals.

The research on suckling ketosis was not well known at the time, and the recommendations were rarely implemented in clinical practice. I raised the issue of suckling ketosis with the consultant neonatologist at the hospital, showing her some of the pilot diaries. These recorded a clear and frequent feeding trail that served to convince her that these babies were getting enough through exclusive breastfeeding. The suckling diary worked a treat with any healthy baby at risk of hypoglycaemia. See Figure 3 on the next page for the pilot suckling diary.

Clinical practice revealed that many mothers suckled their babies for long periods. They often continued at home and shared their experiences through clinics and/or letters. Community midwives and health visitors often telephoned seeking more information. They saw a difference in mothers who spent lots of time holding the baby. Suckling, as defined in the diary, appeared to increase maternal confidence and to restore ownership and control. It appeared to make breastfeeding feel easier – and more instinctive.

During the three years it took to develop the diary, there were many anecdotal clinical experiences of healthy but problem feeders or healthy at-risk babies (moderately preterm, small for gestational age infants, babies of mothers with diabetes) whose mothers were able to breastfeed exclusively using the suckling diary. In 1996, our breastfeeding rates at hospital

Figure 3: Pilot Suckling diary

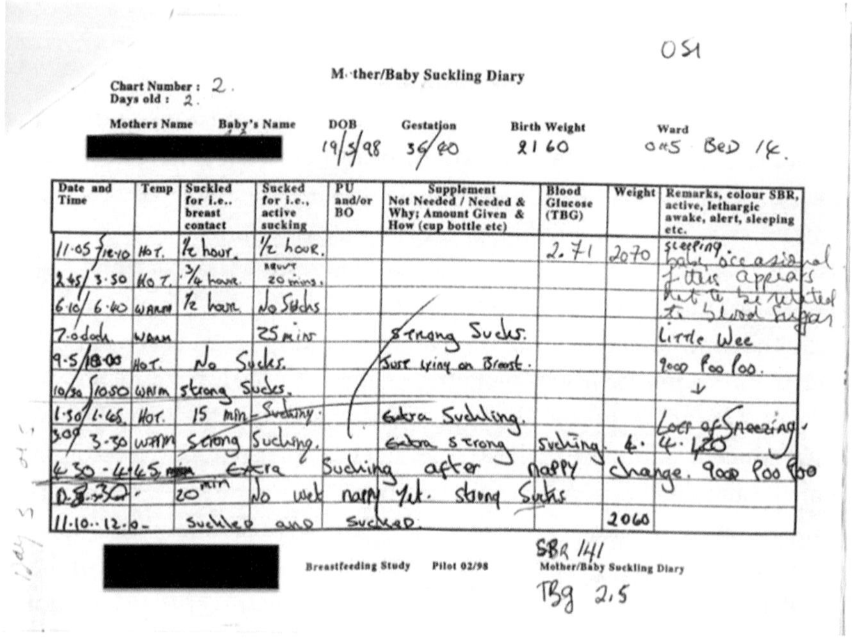

Figure 3: Pilot Suckling diary

discharge were 75%.[13,14] However, the reasons for this success were unclear. While I thought that using the suckling diary was the single most important factor, I continued to observe a number of simple reflex-like movements appearing to stimulate breastfeeding behaviours. And that got me thinking.

Primitive neonatal reflexes develop from around 28 to 32 gestational weeks. At birth the newborn baby has already experienced these movements. In fact, the baby reflexes are a point of continuity from womb to world. I had a sudden light-bulb moment as I realised that there were other points of continuity inherent in BN helping babies to transition from gestational life to neonatal life. Continuity was a key theory supporting the practice of biological nurturing.

CHAPTER 4

The Biological Nurturing Continuum

Continuity is the theoretical heart of biological nurturing. The mammary gland is programmed to take over from the placenta. There is only one requirement: mothers and babies need to remain together, in close physical contact during the early days and weeks. However, in our industrialised cultures, giving birth and breastfeeding are characterised by separation, rupture, and discontinuity.

Continuity and discontinuity are opposing perspectives to explain how infants and children grow and develop. I borrow the terminology from psychology texts to enhance understanding of why biological nurturing works.

Continuity theorists suggest that growth and development are relatively smooth, steady, regular processes, without a distinct beginning or ending. Advocates, mostly behavioural psychologists, argue that many aspects of human development build upon past experiences so that growth is cumulative.[1] However, notions of continuity are currently invisible in the breastfeeding context. For example, we seldom relate breastfeeding to womb feeding. Once I realised the continuum between foetal and neonatal positions, reflexes, and states, I often used continuity theory to support mothers.

It was a real turning point for me when I understood how the development of motion in the womb leads to early neonatal capacity for locomotion that aids latch. Likewise, the foetal "indeterminate" sleep states continue to dominate postnatal behaviours and influence feeding frequency. I felt it was crucial to share these theories with mothers, highlighting the physiological sense implicit in nature's blueprint.

Nature also has a blueprint for mothers. Gradually, I realised that my postnatal support needed to be similar to my role as a midwife accompanying mothers during pregnancy and labour. I didn't need to manage breastfeeding but rather I needed to manage an oxytocin friendly environment conducive to breastfeeding. My clinical practice and research observations suggested there was a nurturing continuum of neonatal and maternal behaviours from womb to world and from pregnancy to immediate postpartum and the postnatal period. Biological nurturing highlights these golden nuggets of continuity hidden within five of its six components (see Figure 4).

These progressive concepts explain why BN works, contrasting with the current gold standard of lactation management. Importantly, these BN variables are behaviours: they're actions or reactions, things that you can see or hear and therefore can describe objectively and reliably. In that way, understanding the biological nurturing continuum helps you explain the rationale to mothers and to your colleagues.

Continuity in Baby Positions

As soon as you practise BN, you find great versatility in the baby's position. This versatility is associated with two BN positional subcomponents: *neonatal lie* (the direction of the baby's position) and *neonatal attitude* (the degree of flexion). Both are mirror images of foetal lie and attitude, maintaining positional continuity from womb to world. Indeed, I was inspired to use these terms in the postnatal context by midwifery prenatal assessments.[2] Notably, foetal lie and attitude, assessed and documented

Figure 4: Continuity of Biological Nurturing Variables

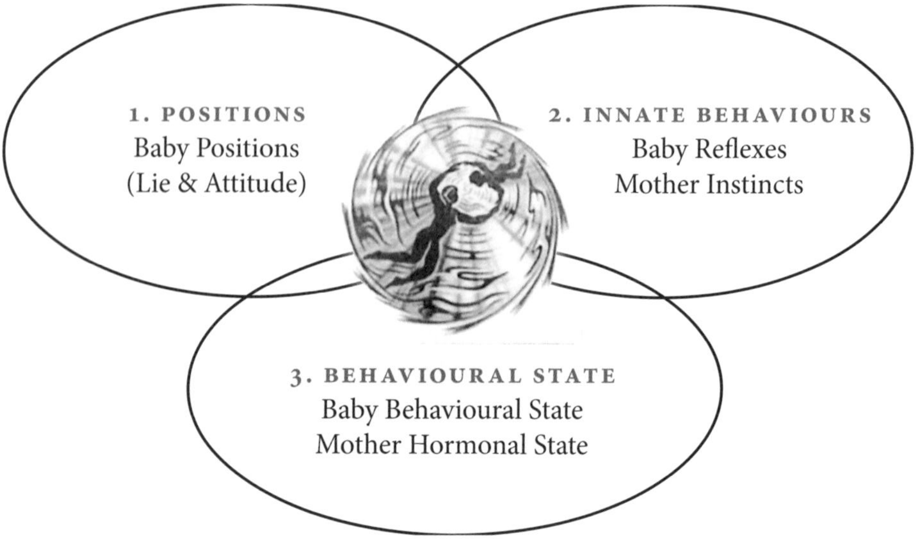

1. POSITIONS
Baby Positions
(Lie & Attitude)

2. INNATE BEHAVIOURS
Baby Reflexes
Mother Instincts

3. BEHAVIOURAL STATE
Baby Behavioural State
Mother Hormonal State

during the third gestational trimester, are strong indicators of how the newborn will spontaneously approach the breast.[3]

Once defined, anyone can observe and describe these two variables objectively and at a glance. From a BN perspective, these positional subcomponents are your first point of assessment anytime mothers experience problems. Neonatal lie and attitude ensure what I call "good fit" and are integral to the BN breastfeeding assessment. We examine how these subcomponents interrelate and interact to aid latch in Chapter 11.

This positional flexibility means that there's not one "correct" way to practise biological nurturing. However, research observations highlight some positional commonalities. First, mothers don't hold their babies in a way that applies pressure along the baby's back, head, or neck. While some mothers grasp baby's bottom, others just make a little nest with their arms around the baby.

Second, the baby always lies prone (on his tummy) but tilted on top of his mother's body. The baby never lies flat and prone, which is a position strongly associated with sudden infant death.[4,5,6]

Third, the front part of baby's entire body always faces and touches mum's body. This means that the baby's thighs, calves, and feet tops can brush up against mum. When they practise BN, many mothers spontaneously support the soles of their baby's feet with their hands or a blanket.

Fourth, this close body apposition, tummy on mummy, means that there is constant abdominal (ventral) contact between mother and baby.

The first three observations are directly related to the mechanisms of biological nurturing and will be discussed in depth in Chapter 8. However, people often ask me why continuous ventral contact is important. Continuous ventral or tummy contact between mother and baby releases navel radiation, a mechanism central to kinetic theories explaining how motion develops during gestation.[7] Masgutova, an expert in reflex integration, calls these movements core limb flexion and extension.[8,9]

In the weightlessness of the womb, floating in an amniotic sea, the foetus receives a constant supply of glucose via the placenta and umbilical cord. During womb feeding, the navel is the nurturing centre, source of attachment, nourishment, and elimination, constantly renewing energy for growth and development. In other words, the navel is the "axis mundi" from which human limbs develop.[10]

Bainbridge, an expert in mind-body centring, suggests that navel radiation is the dominant pattern of foetal movement that ripples out from the centre (the navel) to the limbs and back again in patterns comparable to the radial symmetry found in the starfish.[11]

In utero, as the baby grows, her movements are at first confined and then constrained within the womb. At birth, everything changes. Gravitational forces suddenly exert downward pressure in a cold, bright, open, exposed world without limits or boundaries. The baby's nervous system is immature and initial movements are involuntary and poorly controlled.[12]

When you place an awake and alert newborn on her back, you will likely observe erratic arm and leg cycling or what Prechtl, a well-known Dutch neonatologist, calls spontaneous general movements, describing them as "writhing".[13] Importantly, writhing increases in strength and amplitude as the baby progresses to fussy and crying states. Goddard-Blythe, a freelance consultant in neurodevelopmental education, writes that when you place the same baby prone, lying flat on her tummy, "she will initially squirm and wriggle like a beached fish or worm".[14]

Traditional neurological assessments, such as the Brazelton method – the Neonatal Behavioural Assessment Scale (NBAS) – suggest that these early, jerky, or "unbalanced, cogwheel movements" of arms and legs are linked to the immaturity of the central nervous system (CNS).[15] From birth, the baby's brain starts to fine-tune the abundant neural synaptic connections between the upper and lower brain structures.

Habitually, during this time of early postnatal CNS development, mothers, sitting upright, have been taught to suppress jerky reflex response either by swaddling their babies or restraining baby's arms or legs. Both strategies work by containing the baby's erratic motor activity, which explains why, Inch,[16] who limits herself to upright or side-lying postures, continues to promote swaddling to pin baby's arms to his sides. Importantly, when mothers sit upright, tummy pressure is constantly interrupted. This happens because mothers must close the gap between their bodies and their baby's body, which is exhausting to do throughout an entire breastfeed. My observations of mothers practising BN suggest that the laid-back gradient supporting mum's soft body curves smooth these involuntary jerky reflexes when baby's body is nestled in close.[17] It is likely that sustained close ventral contact naturally soothes baby's tremulous arm and leg cycling reflexes because it releases navel radiation, organising rippling to and from the navel to extremities, promoting fluency in motion.

But there is more! The rippling causes the baby's arms, legs, and feet tops to brush up or rub against mum's body. Body brushing releases motor reflexes, such as placing, arm and leg cycling, stepping, and crawling. Einspieler and Prechtl state that writhing movements dominate for about

6 to 8 weeks of the baby's life, suggesting that neonatal movement remains navel-centric during this time.[18] Interestingly, this corresponds to the time it often takes to establish breastfeeding. Taken together these BN observations suggest that continuity in locomotion or the ability to move easily from one place to another is enhanced by a gradient providing constant ventral tummy to mummy contact.

Continuity in Baby Reflexes

Neonatal navel radiation builds upon and develops further the patterns of foetal movement, but locomotion is closely associated with the expression of smooth primitive neonatal reflexes (PNRs). Archaic or primitive neonatal reflexes are inborn, involuntary reactions to environmental or endogenous stimuli and they develop in utero from around 28 weeks gestation. [19,20]

For many babies, by 34 gestational weeks, the foetal reflex movements are sufficiently mature to aid latch and sustain milk transfer. This is important for late preterm babies. With support and biological nurturing, many of these babies in our study breastfed exclusively from birth. This important point of the continuity characterising BN will be illustrated and discussed further in Chapter 9.

Continuity in Neonatal Behavioural State

We all know that the foetus grows and develops in an environment where conditions remain consistently warm, wet, and dark. But what about foetal behavioural state? Does the foetus remain constantly awake or constantly asleep?

Researchers, such as Nijhuis and his colleagues, set out to answer this question in the 1980s.[21] Using ultrasound together with observations of infants born preterm, they found that the foetus does not remain in one consistent state. The ultrasound traces that you find in the research reports curiously resemble a cardiotocograph (CTG) showing both wake and sleep foetal states using many of the same observable behavioural markers that Brazelton, a well-known American paediatrician, used to define neonatal behavioural states in the 1960s.[22]

The foetus sleeps for about 18 hours a day; because transitions from state to state are irregular and rapid, most of time the baby is in an "indeterminate" light sleep or drowsy state lacking clear definition. Deep sleep develops late during gestation, around 36 weeks.

At birth, mirroring foetal life, the healthy term neonate spends up to three-quarters of her day largely in indeterminate sleep and often has difficulty attaining deep sleep. Therefore, indeterminate sleep states continue to predominate for the first six to eight weeks of neonatal life).[23,24]

Traditionally, mothers have been advised to wait until the baby is in a quiet alert state to breastfeed; even though many babies make sucking movements in their sleep, medical and midwifery experts, and most professional and mainstream breastfeeding books either state that the sleeping baby will not feed or suggest that the baby needs to indicate readiness, i.e., be "visually attentive" to breastfeed.[25,26,27,28]

In contrast, maintaining continuity of indeterminate sleep from foetus to neonate is central to the practice of biological nurturing. Mothers are encouraged to keep their sleeping newborns cheek to breast on their bodies in BN positions. People often react with surprise, asking me: "Why would anyone do that? Why place a sleeping baby on the breast?" The answer is easy. Babies latch on and feed well in light sleep and drowsy states. Unfortunately, most breastfeeding mothers discover this too late to use sleep states to overcome early difficulties. Breastfeeding the sleeping baby is integral to the practice of biological nurturing and we discuss neonatal behavioural states and their BN mechanisms in depth in Chapter 14.

In summary, the biological nurturing continuum emphasises links – robust associations between the baby's position and state from womb to world. These strong relationships help to explain why BN works. They also suggest that practising BN for at least the first 72 hours, the time of metabolic adaptation, may increase breastfeeding duration.

A nurse who attended a presentation I gave in Normandy, France, investigated this hypothesis in 2016. As part of a national lactation diploma, Gadroy carried out a randomised controlled trial comparing BN with standard breastfeeding support in a rural public hospital.[29] In that hospital, despite compliance with the Baby Friendly Ten Steps, including at least one hour of skin-to-skin contact at birth, almost 62% of mothers bottle feed at hospital discharge compared with 38% breastfeeding (32% exclusive).

Focusing on mothers with infants having latching problems on the second postnatal day, Gadroy hypothesised that BN would increase breastfeeding duration. She randomised 32 babies whose mothers intended to breastfeed exclusively for at least six weeks, 16 in each group. Following intervention, no mother in the BN group weaned her baby the first week compared with nine controls. By the end of the second week, four more controls had stopped breastfeeding compared to five mothers in the BN group.

At the end of the first month, these numbers had not changed; 19% of the controls were breastfeeding ($n=3$, 2 exclusively) compared to 69% ($n=11$, 10 exclusively) in the BN group. In this small study, practising BN increased breastfeeding duration significantly. Further research is needed with larger sample sizes.

Nevertheless, the data was interesting, suggesting that by the end of the first two weeks, early unintended breastfeeding cessation may level off as no mother in either group stopped breastfeeding after the second week. One interpretation is related to maturation. The older the baby gets, the more capable she becomes, increasingly able to organise purposeful, smooth movement.

Mothers are often told to persevere with breastfeeding because it gets easier. These results suggest that those mothers who "persevere" using traditional upright and side-lying positions might benefit immediately during the early weeks if they were informed of the BN continuum.

Continuity for Mothers

Giving birth is also fraught with change for the mother. During pregnancy, mothers carry their babies constantly. It would be silly to suggest that they put them down. However, as soon as the baby is born, the mother is advised to keep the baby in a cot or bassinet by her bed. Clinical and anecdotal experiences suggest that many mothers feel "empty" following birth. De Gasquet, a French maternity doctor, suggests that the act of giving birth opens the maternal pelvis and that mothers often experience anxiety because the womb, now empty, needs closure.[30]

Biological nurturing used as a bridging strategy minimises early maternal/neonatal separation and may help with physical or psychological closure. The nurturing/nurturance role of the maternal body that so strongly underpins BN is made explicit, inviting acknowledgement of a simultaneous symbiotic/separation paradox. While practising BN, mothers may not feel so empty after birth; they also may not feel a need to debrief.

A maternal hormonal state associated with high oxytocin pulsatility releases spontaneous breastfeeding behaviours. An oxytocin complexion and innate breastfeeding behaviours are the two other BN components linking pregnancy and postpartum. Continuity underpins both. Maintaining this continuity often helps to ease mothers into their new role (see Figure 4 above).

Continuity of Maternal Hormonal State

Biological nurturing can provide continuity for mothers, specifically in regard to mothers' oxytocin pulsatility. Oxytocin is released both centrally and peripherally before and after birth with maternal blood concentrations rising during the third trimester of pregnancy.[31,32] Oxytocin must be released in a pulsatile fashion to trigger spontaneity. Nissen and her colleagues[33] have shown that oxytocin pulsatility is higher in the first hour following birth than at any other time.

Oxytocin is known as the contraction and ejection hormone. High maternal concentrations may, first and foremost, be a protective mechanism, keeping the uterus well contracted, thus decreasing the risk of primary (first 24 hours after birth) postpartum haemorrhage.[34]

High oxytocin pulsatility on the second postnatal day has also been associated with longer breastfeeding duration.[35] Taken together, this research evidence suggests that the first six weeks is a time of transition. Practising BN for the first six weeks may increase and prolong high oxytocin pulsatility. This would logically lead to increased breastfeeding duration, as well as offering further protection against secondary (the first six postnatal weeks) postpartum haemorrhage. Six weeks is also the time that corresponds to the establishment of lactation and initial CNS maturation.

Biological Nurturing: Keeping Mothers and Babies Together

Biological nurturing respects nature's plan, keeping the baby in the right place at the right time – what Alberts and Cramer[36] termed the right "habitat." Following on from their seminal work, I call this "keeping the baby at the right address." This maintains continuity – familiar voice, heartbeat, odour, and body space for the baby – and sustains maternal oxytocin pulsatility, releasing spontaneous mothering and breastfeeding behaviours. It can also help relieve any separation anxiety or feelings of emptiness the mother might experience. In the early days and weeks, keeping the baby at the right address is an integral part of why biological nurturing works.

CHAPTER 5

Keep the Baby at the Right Address

Alberts and Cramer coined the terms "habitat" and "niche" in the mammalian developmental context over 30 years ago.[1,2] From a psychobiological perspective, Alberts suggested that "learning is not separable from a behaving body." Learning occurs best within "developmental habitats" like the "uterus, the mother's body, and her lactational apparatus".[3] Alberts defines habitat as a location, in space and in time, a life-support system providing ambient temperature, humidity, light, and energy. Simply put, habitat is the baby's "address".[4]

"Niche," on the other hand, is what mammals do in the habitat. In developmental terms, niche is the job of growing up: how the foetus, neonate, infant, juvenile, and adult learn and adapt. Alberts calls this "making a living." The metaphor is apt: each address corresponds to a stage of development, characterised by a different niche or "occupation" that enables the mammal to survive.[5] For the neonate, activities like suckling, mobilising, sleeping, and elimination are part of the learning that we cannot separate from the behaving body of the maternal habitat.

Biological nurturing is a prime example of this perspective, providing stability of the baby's habitat from womb to world. Inside or outside, it's the same address and the newborn nestles amidst familiar sounds, odours, and behaviours. The boundaries are still there, offering warmth, shelter, and protection, but they no longer restrict growth as they did towards the end of gestation.

During the first postnatal days, the time of metabolic adaptation, our priority is to maintain continuity of womb feeding frequency. Obviously, we can never replicate constant placental nutrition, but we can bridge the upcoming and inevitable transition into extrauterine patterns of feeding and fasting. Mothers do that by being proactive; they take the lead, placing their sleeping babies at the right address.

The right address is species-specific and for human babies it's suckling on mother's breast or sleeping cheek to breast. Nurturing the sleeping baby, cheek to breast, is one of the most important aspects of the biological nurturing continuum, offering the opportunity for small, frequent, and sometimes non-stop mammary feeds. That's why I often call biological nurturing a bridging strategy. BN, used as a bridge, helps newborns achieve metabolic adaptation.[6]

Having been passively fed with a constant supply of glucose via the placenta during intrauterine life, healthy term infants are born well fed. At birth, when the umbilical cord ceases to pulsate, this constant energy influx abruptly stops. The neonate must maintain normal blood glucose concentrations while adapting to the feasting/fasting patterns of extrauterine life).[7,8]

Research evidence indicates an association between longer feeding intervals and lower blood glucose concentrations, putting many babies at risk of neonatal hypoglycaemia.[9,10,11] Keeping baby at the right address reduces this risk, shortening the interval between feeds.[12,13] We examine the metabolic transition in greater depth in the next chapter. However, the following case study summarises how we used BN as a bridge for a group of healthy late preterm babies during metabolic research projects in London hospitals.

Research Case Study

My colleagues and I reported how keeping late preterm babies at the right address increased rates of exclusive breastfeeding.[14] During research projects looking at metabolic adaptation for a group of vulnerable babies, one participating mother of an infant born at 34 gestational weeks practised BN with her baby at the right address for 16 of the first 24 hours. Both mother and baby were lightly dressed during that time, not in skin-to-skin contact. Her preterm baby, who would have normally been transferred to special care and tube-fed for the first postnatal hours/days, maintained her temperature and blood glucose concentrations within normal limits throughout and was exclusively breastfed from birth to over 4 months, which was the primary outcome measure.

Proximity Matters

Today in most hospitals in the industrialised world, mothers are encouraged to keep their babies, at arm's length, in a cot that resembles a plastic box (see Figure 5).

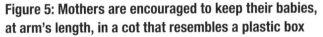

Figure 5: Mothers are encouraged to keep their babies, at arm's length, in a cot that resembles a plastic box

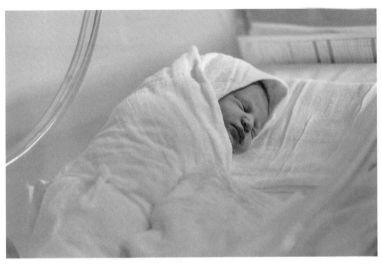

Many health professionals, and mothers alike, think that newborn babies should sleep in that box between feeds. In our cultures, the plastic box, furnished by the hospital and kept close to mum's bed, underpins an early mothering style called rooming-in.

What is Rooming-In?

Introduced in the 1940s as a part of a return to a more natural paradigm where mothers were not separated from their babies at birth, rooming-in was a major breakthrough. Rooming-in brought mothers and babies closer together. This immediately increased breastfeeding rates despite long intervals when baby slept at arm's length. This form of early contact still works well for many mothers, especially those who have what I like to call "book babies" or those babies who do exactly what experts have written in the childcare books.

For those who don't have "book babies," the separation implicit with keeping baby at arm's length often creates a breastfeeding struggle. This leads us to highlight erroneous assumptions associated with rooming-in. Look at

Figure 6: Unlike human babies, lower-brained and hoofed mammals mobilise rapidly and independently at birth

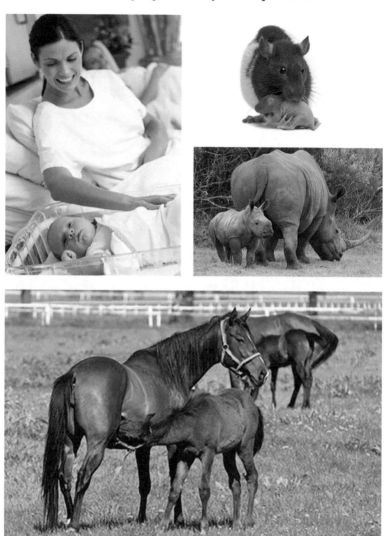

Figure 6. Do you see that our current rooming-in practices correspond to the maternal habitat of mammals that display independent niche-learning activities? These animals, such as the lower-brained and hoofed mammals, mobilise freely at birth and feed independently. Apparently, rodents and hoofed mammalian mothers don't actively initiate or participate in these activities. Rather they appear to rely upon the baby to take the lead. Unlike baby rats and ungulates, it is not in the repertoire of our babies to move great distances or quickly from one place to another. These simple observations

concerning neonatal motor skills appear to be greatly misunderstood among those health professionals who promote skin-to-skin contact and responsive or baby-led breastfeeding. We discuss myths associated with baby-led feeding in Chapter 6, but examining beliefs and practices associated with skin-to-skin contact takes precedence.

Limitations of Skin-to-Skin Contact

Much like biological nurturing, skin-to-skin contact is a form of early mother baby interaction that ensures continuity from womb to world. During the past 20 years, research has suggested that naked mother–baby contact is the independent or causative variable increasing breastfeeding initiation.[15]

Skin-to-skin contact can be a wonderful practice. Unfortunately, this is often poorly applied and can undermine mothers' confidence. There are two main concerns I have noted. The first is that practitioners often misapply research on the breast crawl, making it difficult for both mother and baby. The second concern, which I addressed briefly in Chapter 2, relates to mothers' control over their amount of exposure and nudity.

The breast crawl research has captivated the hearts of mothers and professionals alike. However, close scrutiny reveals that many babies do not actually latch on and breastfeed during periods of extended birth skin-to-skin contact as illustrated in the following findings of a frequently cited study.

Study Review

Widström and her colleagues[16] placed 28 babies in skin-to-skin contact between their mothers' breasts with their eyes at nipple level during the first postnatal hour. Mothers were asked NOT to shift baby's position or help them find the breast. The objective was to describe behavioural sequences leading to self-attachment and nine phases were identified. The birth cry (intense crying lasting from two to four minutes) was followed by relaxation, awakening and activity, where babies moved a lot without shifting their position. Following these four phases, 25 babies (89% of the sample) needed to rest, after which seven (25%) were still unable to shift their position (crawling phase).

Ten babies (36%) couldn't move independently from between their mother's breasts to the areola (the primary outcome). Of those 18 who did, three were too tired to suckle and, once they had arrived, it took up to 45 minutes for the others to self-attach. By 120 minutes all babies were sound asleep. Following 120 minutes of skin-to-skin contact, only 15 babies (slightly more than half the sample) actually breastfed.

Widström and Colleagues' Interpretations

The researchers explain that many "babies worked hard to locate the breast" and required a time-out or resting phase. "Infants should not be pushed to go on searching while resting but be left in peace." It is unwise for mothers to "help the infant to attach because, unfortunately, their help sometimes forces the baby. The infant may experience suffocation, fight the breast, and establish aversive behaviours when later coming close to the breast." This interpretation concurs with their Swedish colleague Lennart Righard's beliefs that babies breastfeed, not mothers.[17]

Biological Nurturing Interpretations

When almost half of a research sample does not achieve the primary outcome measure during two hours of close, naked, ventral contact, we need to ask why those 13 babies didn't latch. The immediate answer is easy; because the mothers were not allowed to place and help them, those 13 babies were not at the right address early enough! But there are other issues leading us to critically appraise the research assumptions and procedures.

Is Skin-to-Skin Contact a Habitat?

Health professionals often assume that skin-to-skin contact is a habitat, yet Alberts and Cramer never mention the words. They never state that it is necessary or integral to the "spatial location" of any mammalian learning body. This is probably because skin-to-skin contact is not an address. Rather, it is a dress state describing the presence or absence of clothing. The right breastfeeding address has everything to do with location and little to do with what you wear.

A second assumption concerns the right place on the mother's body. The right "spatial location" for human breastfeeding is NOT just anywhere on the mother's chest or abdomen. As stated above, the right place is either sleeping cheek-to-breast or suckling, defined as licking, mouthing, rooting, and nutritive and non-nutritive sucking. Figure 7 illustrates the right breast-feeding address and some of the wrong places in which health professionals frequently position babies to breastfeed.

The Right Breastfeeding Address

Many practitioners ask: "What's wrong with placing a baby between her mother's breasts, or high up under her chin or low down on her abdomen?" Nothing, really. They're just not optimal for breastfeeding. There are three lines of research that support having babies at the right breastfeeding address.

Figure 7: The Right Address: Always on the Mother's Breast

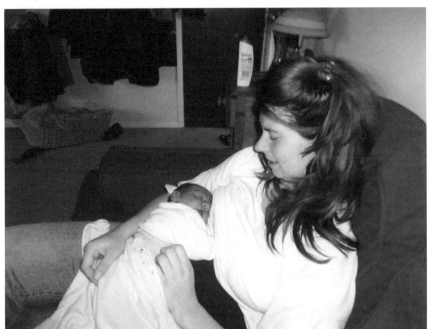

Either sleeping cheek to breast...

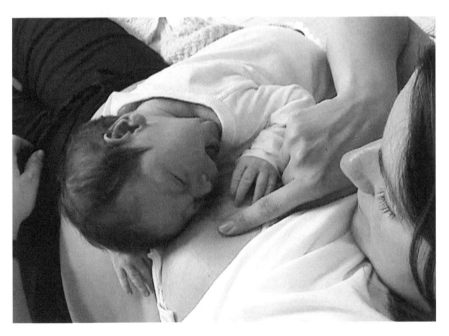

Or latching cheek to breast...

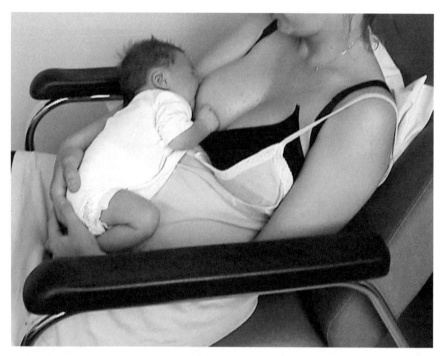

Or actively transferring milk asleep or awake...

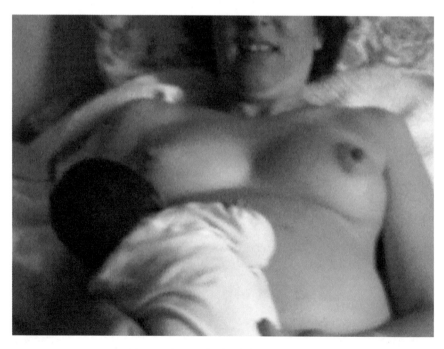

Not on the mother's abdomen...

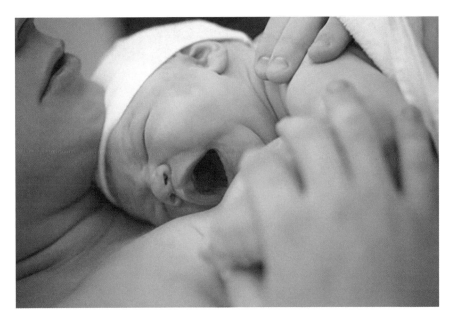

Not under her chin...

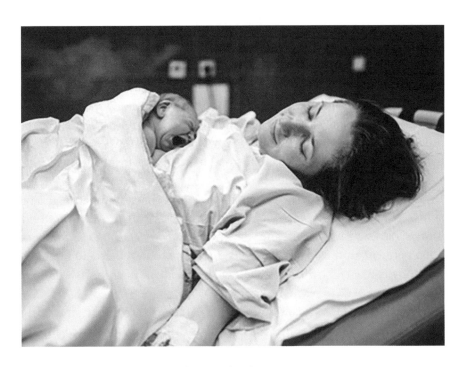

Not between her breasts...

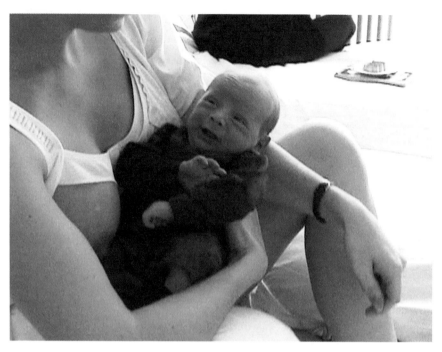

Not in her arms...

First, we know that 80% of mothers spontaneously place and carry their babies with their heads lying on the left breast, and this has nothing to do with being right or left-handed.[18] This left-sided preference is often interpreted as a natural way to calm and comfort the baby because he hears mum's rhythmic heartbeat. However, it's also an example of a maternal instinctual breastfeeding behaviour that makes it easy for the baby to find the breast, latch on, and feed.

Second, we know that the human neonate is born with immature motor skills. At birth, *Homo sapiens* can't turn around or turn over. Desmond Morris, the English zoologist and well known baby watcher, notes: "Mothers must perform all the physical actions that serve to keep her and her baby in bodily contact".[19] Unlike hoofed or lower-brained mammals, a human adult always needs to place the baby.

In the last chapter, we saw how experts paint a negative portrait of early neonatal movement. Prechtl describes "writhing" and Goddard-Blythe compares the baby's movements to "squirming and wriggling of worms or beached fish." It is noteworthy that these observations are made when babies are either placed prone or on their backs; in both positions the baby lies horizontally on a flat surface. When babies are placed prone and flat in a cot, on an examination table, or a fully recumbent maternal body, like in Widström's study, locomotion is challenged. Lying flat exacerbates those writhing, wriggling movements because there's no support or base for baby's feet and no surface resistance. This makes it difficult for the baby to shift the position of his trunk.

Healthy term babies have an inborn forward drive. In Widström's study, mothers were placed lying flat on their backs. There was no gradient providing foot support to help the babies push up. These mechanisms may explain why almost half of the babies failed to reach the mother's areola. In other words, those jerky, erratic movements got those babies nowhere fast.

In contrast, the maternal body slope in biological nurturing positions always provides an escalating base. In BN, three primitive neonatal foot reflexes help a baby climb up her mother's body: *the placing reflex* enables the baby to step up; *the plantar grasp reflex,* and *the sustained Babinski toe fan* stabilise baby's position as she pushes upward. These reflexes anchor movement, aiding forward locomotion. These reflexes were not included in Widström's study, probably because there was no natural foot support. This may also explain why so many of the babies did not reach the areola (the primary outcome measure). There's a strong association between these three foot reflexes and latch.

The mere expression of the upward movement is as important as actually shifting the trunk of the body forward. During biological nurturing, babies are already on the breast; their calves and thighs push upward with imperceptible changes in mouth-to-breast position.

Babies easily move their heads from side to side but rarely shift their trunks or torsos backwards, which explains why placing the baby under the mother's chin makes it nearly impossible for a baby to self-attach. Mum will often need to move her baby down onto the breast.

Third, when health professionals place the baby on the mother's abdomen and then instruct the mother not to shift the baby's position, the neonate must move quite a distance (maybe six, eight, or ten inches) before reaching the breast and then some two to three inches before reaching the areola. This is another unhelpful misapplication of the breast-crawl literature and leads us to ask an important question.

How Long Does It Normally Take a Baby to Find the Breast and Latch?

Well, that answer depends upon the location of the baby. When babies are placed between their mother's breasts in skin-to-skin contact, we know that they take on average 55 minutes to self-attach, having moved two to three inches at most.[20] In the above study that time was doubled.[21]

In real time, this actually feels quite long. However, apart from the skin-to-skin studies, few researchers have looked at latching times. In the biological nurturing study, raw data, collected from birth to 30 postnatal days, reveal the mean time to sustained latch was five minutes (range eight seconds to 16 minutes) and over half the babies self-attached. These latching times concur roughly with Bullough's and colleagues' findings in the immediate postpartum.[22] They calculated a mean time of 7.25 minutes (range 3.5 to 15 minutes) from birth to first suckling for a sample of 76 babies who were dried, wrapped, and put to breast within three minutes. Importantly, in both studies, without pushing or forcing, mothers spontaneously shifted babies' positions, helping them latch.

In contrast, in order to establish a "norm" of 55 minutes, skin-to-skin researchers have controlled maternal participation, effectively extrapolating hoofed and lower-brained mammalian maternal feeding behaviours to the human context. This probably slowed babies down. Taken together, these results suggest that mothers' instinctual breastfeeding behaviours are key. Mothers gently help babies find the breast and this greatly reduces latching times.

Biological nurturing emphasises the breastfeeding relationship. It's not a one-person show; two people actively participate. Concurring with Desmond Morris' observations, the act has to be mother-led because mothers must pick their babies up to breastfeed them. During episodes of BN, mothers are encouraged to help as needed. Observations suggest that mothers intuitively make a body nest; protecting their babies, they move them up their bodies, placing them at the right address at the right time. This often leads the baby to self-attach almost immediately. When it doesn't, mothers help spontaneously by releasing the three foot reflexes, forming their nipple, and/or compressing their breast, and gently coordinating the latch. Arguably, the time it takes to latch relies upon spontaneous, reciprocal mother–baby interactions, not upon "babies working hard" in skin-to-skin contact.[23]

Unfortunately, today, in many hospitals it's the health professional who takes the lead by placing the baby on mum's body and latching the baby for the mother.

Interestingly, many mothers recount that the people who are rough, "pushing babies onto the breast," are often the very health professionals who are showing them how to breastfeed. Read one mother's experience:

◆

SHAZIA'S TESTIMONIAL

I always wanted to breastfeed but my baby and I missed out on the first hour in skin-to-skin contact because the midwives wouldn't let me have him. Some time later, another midwife came to help me with breastfeeding but she couldn't get him to latch.

A few hours later two more midwives forced my baby to latch. They kept pushing at his neck and at the back of his head. He couldn't turn his head or move it backwards. His tiny arms were fluttering while he cried so they held his hands tightly and he couldn't move. While one midwife held his hands, the other one put my breast into his mouth while pinching his cheeks and pushing at the back of his neck. I asked: "Is that normal?" He was crying so much I said: "It seems that he doesn't want this and the way you're putting pressure on his neck seems painful." They replied to me that it was totally normal and that he didn't feel discomfort or pain. They said he was just being stubborn and had to learn how to latch and drink. When it didn't work, they just gave him a bottle of formula.

With zero knowledge and a strange feeling in my heart, I let it happen almost every feed for the next few days during my hospital stay. I also used their method myself since I thought that they were the experts.

My baby cried for almost one hour before they gave up and gave him milk I had expressed. Sometimes their method worked and after resisting my baby latched and drank. But most of the time it didn't work.

I was afraid to take my baby home after a few days since the breastfeeding wasn't successful yet. So, the hospital arranged for extra help for one week at home. Most of the time my baby rejected my breast and got upset the moment I took my breast near him. His cries pierced right through my heart.

◆

This hands-on approach, introduced in the 1980s, usurps power and often reduces maternal confidence, leading to feelings of helplessness. Theoretically, midwives are no longer practising in this way. However,

Shazia's experience dates from January 2018, suggesting otherwise.

Disallowing maternal participation raises a final issue. When you restrict maternal spontaneity, as in some of the skin-to-skin studies, the onus for breastfeeding success is placed entirely upon the baby. Even though many babies became exhausted, requiring long periods of rest, the researchers did not question the efficacy of their protocol.

Newborn exhaustion often results from prolonged jerky, erratic reflex movements, intense crying, and long between-feed intervals. Widström and her colleagues considered it normal, even beneficial, for a newborn baby to cry intensively for two to four minutes. It's no wonder that during the first 30 minutes, almost 90% of the babies in their study required extended periods of rest.

Following a gentle, physiological hospital or home birth, many babies vocalise but few cry for extended periods. Following birth, no mother would ever spontaneously lie down on her back and place her baby under her chin or between her breasts with baby's eyes in line with her areolas. That is learned behaviour. When birth is physiological, mothers are often in upright postures. First, they often gaze at their babies, and then they establish eye-to-eye contact and gently touch them.[24]

This myth, expert midwives versus "incompetent" mothers, has permeated our belief systems since the time of Cadogan – even some Baby Friendly hospitals mandate showing mothers how to breastfeed and many midwives continue to take the lead. It is not uncommon to hear a midwife say: "I can't get that baby to latch!" These beliefs lead to broad general claims like this one I received from a lactation consultant highlighting neonatal competence without acknowledging any maternal know-how.

> All babies are born with a survival instinct and will make their way, find the breast and self-attach…eventually. Most mothers get frustrated and in a rush, eager to have the baby feed, they push them onto the breast.

Look at Figure 8. Will any of these newborn babies make their way independently to the breast and self-attach?

These observations explain why biological nurturing is proactive. Mothers are encouraged to take the lead. Mothers are in control: they decide their dress level and they spontaneously place their sleeping babies at the right address: on the breast. Mothers read babies' feeding cues and actively help as needed. Alberts stressed that you cannot separate adaptation and learning from a "behaving body." In BN, the mother's and baby's bodies

Figure 8: These babies won't make their own way to their mother's breast

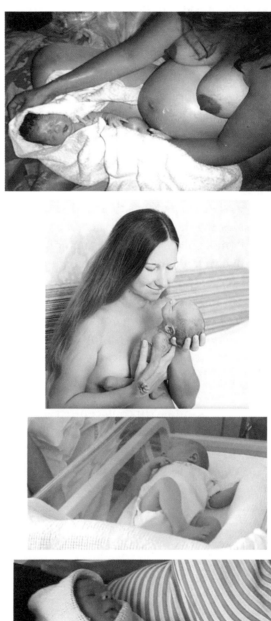

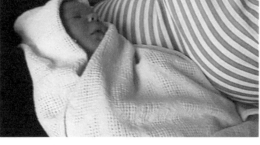

interact. Maternal behaviour is as important as the baby's. Both mother and baby learn from a reciprocal behaving body.

Does This Mean That Mothers Shouldn't Practise Skin-to-Skin Contact?

Skin-to-skin contact is a lovely way to greet the baby at birth. However, our mission is to keep the baby at the address that promotes early suckling. Practising skin-to-skin contact AND biological nurturing during the first postnatal hour is a good combination. Both practices keep mothers and babies together, helping them cope with the discontinuity that inevitably characterises pregnancy, labour, and birth.

Ultimately, dress state is a mother's choice. Mothers are the only experts for their babies, assessing their own and their babies' needs. At birth, our priorities are to promote maternal comfort and dignity by providing an environment conducive to the release of high oxytocin pulsatility, which in turn releases maternal spontaneity and instinctual breastfeeding behaviours. We have been unkind to mothers by suggesting that they should feed their babies like lower-brained and/or hoofed mammals do. We need to place mothers, not just their babies, at the centre of care.

We also need to focus upon mimicking womb feeding frequencies, reducing the interval between giving birth and the first breastfeed. Suggesting that mothers should not participate and waiting for two hours for the baby to latch in skin-to-skin contact often compromises neonatal metabolic adaptation by delaying the first suckling. Biological nurturing is a proactive, mother-centred approach that reduces the time to latch. After birth, mothers should be encouraged to practise BN in as much skin-to-skin contact as they desire. If the baby is at the right address, mothers do not need to be undressed.

CHAPTER 6

Transitions: Coping with Discontinuity

Traditionally, we have viewed birth as a new beginning. As soon as we cut the umbilical cord, we end placental function. The baby has departed the protective intrauterine environment, which was warm, wet, and a dark place where sounds were muffled and space was restricted. Comparatively, the extrauterine environment is cold, dry, bright, and loud. Space is infinite–limitless. Importantly, in the womb, the baby was fed passively, receiving a constant supply of maternal glucose and other nutrients via the umbilical cord. Now the newborn must actively suck for his supper.

Anabolic pathways, such as lipogenesis and glycogenesis, characterise foetal life; glucose was the primary energy substrate and the foetus stocked up, storing fat and glycogen, with a 48-hour reserve.[1] At birth, the baby must cope with discontinuity, switching to a "variable fat-based fuel economy".[2] Glycogenolysis and lipolysis – catabolic pathways – are active, especially during the first two days. The baby breaks down glycogen reserves and fat stored in adipose tissue until more copious breastmilk feeds are established. The metabolic pathways, which enable him to take over independent or endogenous production of glucose, are activated.

Jane Hawdon, a metabolic expert in London, explains that at birth there is normally a sharp fall in blood glucose (BG) concentrations followed by a slow rise from a nadir that occurs during the first 12 hours. She discusses nature's back-up plan. When BG levels are in the lower ranges of normal, the healthy term or moderately preterm baby responds through a process called counterregulation. The baby mobilises alternative fuels such as lactate and ketone bodies.[3] The processes are elegant and finely tuned to ensure what Ward Platt and Deshpande, metabolic experts in Newcastle, sum up as "metabolic and hormonal adaptive changes that ensure a continuing supply of energy fuels and constitute the neonatal metabolic adaptation".[4]

Understanding the physiology involved in the metabolic transition is complex and exceeds the scope of this book. Arguably, a rudimentary understanding of metabolic adaptation should underpin our feeding policies, and therefore I highlight that we are fortunate to have world famous experts in metabolic adaptation in Britain and I heartily recommend that you read their work, together with research and commentaries published by Laura DeRooy and Anthony Williams.

For our purposes, and to support breastfeeding, we must take on board two important issues. First, to ensure a successful metabolic transition, the healthy term infant needs to actively suckle, mimicking womb feeding, ingesting small drops of colostrum frequently. Second, breastfed and artificially fed babies have different patterns of metabolic adaptation. For example, artificial feeding, or any supplementation with non-human breastmilk substitutes, suppresses suckling ketosis with peak ketone body concentrations being inversely proportional to the amount of formula given.[5-10]

In the last chapter, we introduced Albert's theories suggesting that you cannot separate early niche learning from a behaving body: the mother's body is the baby's habitat.[11] Reciprocally, close contact with the baby's behaving body releases instinctive breastfeeding. We also discussed how biological nurturing bridges postnatal transition when mothers keep their babies at the right address.

A plethora of research has examined how labour ward routines often disrupt breastfeeding by separating mothers and babies at birth.[12] Today midwives across the world are aware of the benefits of keeping mothers and babies together in the immediate postpartum.

In contrast, few researchers have examined how some of our most cherished postnatal policies often delay suckling and metabolic adaptation by inadvertently separating mothers and babies from the "behaving body" during the first 48 to 72 hours. The first part of this chapter therefore focuses on a typical postnatal ward scenario during the first two days. In particular, I critically appraise policies that promote responsive breastfeeding and manual expression of colostrum.

Then, I define discontinuity from womb to world with a view to compare and contrast the discontinuous critical time-sensitive viewpoint with the biological nurturing perspective.

Finally, I discuss professional breastfeeding assessment, which is the cornerstone of good practice. To be effective, assessment should be quick and easy to do, characterised by valid and reliable indicators of milk transfer and mother–baby well-being. In this part of the chapter, we differentiate some trustworthy indicators of effective breastfeeding from some traditional but invalid observations that often create maternal fear and anxiety. Fear and anxiety are breastfeeding enemies!

The First 24 Hours

Following a "golden" or "magic hour" of skin-to-skin contact at birth, it is widely accepted that babies sleep. Mother and baby are transferred to the postnatal ward. As said previously, in our industrialised nations, as soon as babies sleep, we often wrap or swaddle them and place them in that plastic cot, rooming-in next to the mother's bed. The babies appear settled, comfortable, and calm, and mothers are told to wait for their newborns to cue, indicating readiness to breastfeed.[13,14] This is part and parcel of responsive breastfeeding.

What is Responsive Breastfeeding?

Responsive breastfeeding is the new buzzword for demand or baby-led feeding. The Academy of Breastfeeding Medicine (ABM) recommends demand feeding at least every three hours.[15] The Public Health Agency defines "readiness" as baby cues or early feeding signals, for example, when baby licks her lips, makes sucking sounds, or sucks her fingers.[16] The UK Baby Friendly Initiative concurs but adds that mothers also need to understand that breastfeeding is a means of comforting and calming babies and themselves.[17]

Interestingly, many mothers feel relieved and serenely calm after birth but too excited to sleep even when they have given birth in the middle of the night. So they often watch their babies, patiently waiting for the feeding cues signalling readiness. Many babies, when placed in the plastic cot, sleep for a very long stretch, maybe six to eight hours. In that case, on the first day, hospital policy often suggests that mothers use gentle rousing techniques to awaken their babies for a breastfeed. When babies fail to latch or refuse the breast, mothers are taught how to hand express their colostrum.

Hand expression has become a real focus of breastfeeding practice during the first 24 hours.[18–20] Expressed colostrum is described as an amazing "gift" and it is given to the baby via a plastic spoon, cup, or syringe.[21] Jane Morton, a paediatrician at Stanford University, recommends that all mothers hand express their colostrum during the first days. She states that "effective removal of small amounts of colostrum will stimulate breastmilk production" because "many babies who are with their mothers need help and time before they learn how to breastfeed effectively." This is illustrated in a lovely video.[22]

Although some mothers can express up to 5 millilitres (mls), most will only express a small amount, as seen in the video clip where Morton advises using a miniscule 1-ml container to collect the colostrum. In fact, research findings suggest that the median amount mothers can express in the early postpartum is one-half of 1 ml (0.5 ml).[23] This is because no artificial method of breastmilk expression can compete with a healthy term baby's sucking action.[24]

Many mothers find hand expression during the first 24 hours frustrating and anxiety producing. Visual acuity is our primary sense. People often say, "seeing is believing." Given the small average quantities, it's no wonder that many mothers think that they haven't got enough milk.[25]

Should Mothers Hand Express Even If They Do Not Have Any Problems?

Today, in the UK Baby-Friendly hospitals, all mothers are taught to hand express their milk before hospital discharge.[26] The UK BFI supports this practice, citing Flaherman and colleagues' randomised trial comparing hand expression with breast pumping for mothers of healthy term newborns.[27] Entwistle writes in the evidence supporting BFI practice that "hand expression in the early postpartum period improves breastfeeding rates at two months for mothers of healthy term babies".[28] However, the target group of this study was babies with latching and sucking difficulties. Flaherman and her colleagues excluded any infant who did not have feeding problems.

The UK BFI standards do not explicitly state that all mothers of healthy term babies should hand express. However, when babies fail to breastfeed despite awakening them and giving support with positioning and attachment, hand expression is the "go-to" strategy. Read the following testimonial I received from a concerned physician.

◆

TESTIMONIAL

Mothers with well babies are taught to express by hand, displacing more natural breastfeeding support. Although they are also supported to latch and nurse their babies, there is a checklist approach to both of these skills which appears to confer upon them equal importance. Moreover, the act of giving a baby a drop of colostrum on the finger is regarded and often recorded as feeding, which can falsely reassure the mother that all is well, and mask the fact that a baby is sick.

◆

In addition, many health professionals believe that hand expression will increase a mother's milk supply. They therefore suggest that all mothers, not just those experiencing problems, hand express after each breastfeed. When Australian researchers asked mothers why they were not feeding directly at the breast, almost half said: "professional advice." Other reasons included attaching and sucking difficulties, having a sleepy baby, not having enough milk, nipple pain and trauma, the infant having a low blood sugar, and staff concern about infant weight loss.[29] This practice has resulted in large numbers of mothers across the industrialised world expressing their milk during the first 48 hours to give breastmilk feeds.[30-35]

What Does the Research Say?

Numerous researchers have looked at the effects of supplementing early active suckling with breastmilk expression. Some studies report that expression increases breastfeeding duration.[36] Others suggest the opposite.[37,38] This mixed bag of evidence prompted Forster and her colleagues in Australia to compare breastfeeding outcomes for women actively suckling their babies, feeding them solely at the breast, with those who also supplemented with either expressed breastmilk (EBM) and/or infant formula. Their findings clearly demonstrate that mothers who actively breastfeed their infants their breastmilk only (with no milk expression) in the first 24–48 hours were more likely to be breastfeeding at six months. Forster and her colleagues conclude that mothers of healthy term infants should be encouraged and supported to feed directly from the breast right from the start.[39]

These findings are in line with my personal beliefs, as well as my results for breastfeeding duration in research projects and clinical practice. Let us now explore some potential interpretations of this phenomenon.

The issues are complex. Theoretically, milk expression is a logical solution. We know that breast emptying creates and maintains milk production and sufficiency. However, from a physiological perspective, for healthy term infants, hand expression may delay the normal progression of lactogenesis. The pumping action involved in milk expression can only mimic the baby's suckling mechanism. The breastfeeding baby releases a hormonal response through active suckling. The hormonal response to expression is not the same.[40]

Active Suckling Matters!

The normal yield during the first 24 hours for healthy mothers actively breastfeeding their healthy term infants is 50 ml.[41] That is a tenfold difference from hand expression. Look at the numbers: if you encourage a mother to hand express eight times during the first 24 hours, she will extract on average 4 ml of colostrum. Our aim is not to routinely increase all mothers' milk secretion in a uniform fashion but rather to keep the baby in the maternal habitat, which enables the baby to "learn from a behaving body" and feed as frequently as he or she needs to individualise her milk supply. But there are other reasons to promote active suckling. First, giving any milk via cup, spoon, or syringe will inevitably disrupt the baby's natural rhythms. Early colostral supplements likely confuse imprinting mechanisms, filling babies up inappropriately; this often increases the interval between early, active latchments.

Latchment is a term introduced by Elsie Mobbs, an Australian midwife.[42] She suggests that the first latchments are imprinting behaviours. Human babies are biologically designed to recognise the breast as a "one-object sucking preference" as opposed to introducing a sucking substitute. Any artificial feeding device, bottle teat, cup, spoon, or finger as the initial or dominant sucking experience, imprints on the baby a psychological and physiological response that often interferes with active breast suckling. This has been called "decoy feeding" where a baby becomes imprinted to a breast substitute that may become his feeding preference. Mobbs suggests that once imprinted, the baby may experience emotional distress on the loss of such stimulus.

Early frequent latchments imprint the baby to the breast sooner. They also maintain some continuity of feeding frequency from womb to world thus reducing the interval between mammary feeds. Long between-feed intervals during the first week do not mimic womb feeding and are not productive for any healthy newborn. Importantly, the earlier healthy term babies actively suckle and swallow, the more they can.

Second, artificial milk extraction likely changes the composition of early colostrum. The active components of colostrum evolve from feed to feed, sometimes during the same feed. The more the baby actively suckles, the quicker the colostrum transitions into mature milk. This means that each baby receives his or her full complement of colostrum.

Third, in view of the inevitable low maternal hand expressed output, many hospital midwives worry about neonatal hypoglycaemia, and they often feel obliged to add artificial milk drink (infant formula) to complement this meagre amount. This addition, in fact, eliminates the neonate's endogenous counterregulatory mechanisms, such as lactate and suckling ketosis, which protect him from hypoglycaemia. In other words, the intervention can cause the pathology it aspires to eliminate.

Mothers' colostrum is rich in fats with a small amount of carbohydrate compared to non-human breastmilk substitutes. The high fat content in mothers' initial colostrum supports the net shift from glucose to fat that characterises metabolic adaptation. Giving the baby regular complements of any breastmilk substitute keeps the baby in an anabolic state resembling foetal life where the baby was passively fed with glucose dominance.

In a rebound effect, increasing neonatal carbohydrate intake maintains that insulin-dominant foetal environment, delaying metabolic handover to glucagon, an important hormone in the regulation of normal glucose concentrations.

Furthermore, hand expression during the first 48 hours removes babies from the habitat of the learning body.[43] The baby is fed passively. My clinical experience suggests that many such babies, returned to mothers' arms, are slow to find the breast even when they are nipple to nose. Many such babies experience difficulty coordinating sucking and swallowing with breathing.

Milk expression also removes mothers from the habitat of the learning body. The act of breastfeeding is body-to-body learning. Hand expression keeps the baby at arm's length. Maternal oxytocin pulsatility is not the same when expressing compared to active suckling.[44] Physiologically, the first 24 to 72 hours after birth are primed by oxytocin. Learning how to hand express stimulates thinking, decreasing oxytocin. This may cause mothers to worry, hesitate, or postpone the suckling act. Milk expression likely removes all the joy of breastfeeding! Arguably, an instinctive act has been transformed into a learned, passive medical process.

Even when a healthy term baby needs to be separated from her mum for a few minutes or for several hours, it's not helpful to immediately teach her how to hand express colostrum. Not only does the healthy term baby arrive in the world well fed but she has reserves covering her first 48 hours.

Finally, it must be said that there are some cost issues. Many hospital administrators and policy makers believe that encouraging all mothers to hand express will promote early discharge. This frees beds. From the hospital's perspective, breastfeeding is often considered a feeding method, like bottle feeding, a way to provide a meal, which is the hospital's statutory duty for all patients. Many hospitals are reluctant to discharge babies until they're gaining weight. The hospital rationale is that filling babies up with hand expressed colostrum will make them settle and gain weight sooner. The reality is that many babies start gaining because they have received a mix of colostrum and artificial milk drink, which makes the baby sleep longer, mimicking a settled state, increasing the interval between feeds.

Typically, many healthy term babies sleep "calmly and quietly," spending the best part of the first 24 hours at arm's length, settled in the plastic cot, separated from mother despite being in the same room.

The Second 24 Hours

The ABM define babies "feeding well" as those babies who awaken the next day, eager to establish two to three hourly demand feeds.[45] The reality is that babies who haven't been located at the right address on the first day have missed out on all that early niche body learning.

During the second postnatal day, many babies either remain sleepy when mothers attempt to breastfeed or they fight the breast. In either case, the baby continues to have spoon or cup feeds of expressed colostrum supplemented by artificial milk drink.

As the learning deficit increases, the fat and glycogen reserves decrease. Counterregulation has been suppressed since yesterday. Morton does not suggest supplementing expressed colostrum with human milk substitutes. However, many hospital midwives do this routinely. As soon as babies show signs of gaining weight, everyone's happy. Mum is often discharged home, "breastmilk feeding exclusively" even though the baby has never actively breastfed.

This perspective, fraught with received ideas and culturally accepted mother–baby separation, is the dominant way of thinking, the way health professionals are taught, and the way mothers are usually taught during antenatal education. Importantly, it characterises discontinuous theories of baby growth and development.

What is Discontinuity?

Discontinuity is a child development term. Experts such as the Swiss psychologist Piaget suggest that human growth, for example, the development of cognition, occurs in distinct stages. Each stage is progressive because one or two tasks must be accomplished before the next stage can start. Like metamorphosis, each stage has a change in habitat and behaviour. Once a stage is complete, you move on and never look back.

Pregnancy, birth and lactation are prime examples of discontinuity. Traditionally, they are reduced to distinct and separate stages: embryonic and foetal growth and development start and finish during trimesters of pregnancy. Pregnancy ends when the baby is born, following three distinct stages of labour that end when the cord is severed and the placenta delivered. Lactogenesis is defined as a two or sometimes three-stage process. Importantly, discontinuous theory suggests that critical and sensitive periods order growth and development within each stage.

Discontinuous Perspectives: The First Hour Following Birth

Like Piaget's theories of cognitive development, all discontinuous approaches mandate a critical, sensitive period during which time you need to accomplish at least one task before moving on to the next stage. Although some experts prefer the term "sensitive" period, it is often argued that the first hour following birth is a golden or magical time when it's "critical" to bond and commence breastfeeding.[46,47] This is why the BFI mandates skin-to-skin contact immediately after birth, lasting until the first successful breastfeed.[48] And yes, that does make physiological sense! Many mothers and babies are particularly sensitive and hormonally synchronised to ease into breastfeeding at this time, especially those who have had straightforward, natural births without any analgesia or intervention. As long as mothers are not taught or shown how to breastfeed, being with the baby, body-to-body, as soon as possible after birth often increases their confidence in their innate capacity.

Nevertheless, many mothers and babies are not immediately ready for bonding. Pharmaceutical pain relief during labour, unexpected caesarean section, fear, embarrassment, and exhaustion are just five factors that can mask maternal sensitivity in the immediate postpartum. For some of these mothers, remaining in skin-to-skin contact for one or two hours (that is until the baby achieves a successful breastfeed or sleeps) might set the bar too high. For example, subdued maternal sensitivity and instructions not to assist the baby may explain why almost half the sample did not reach the areola (the primary outcome measure) in skin-to-skin contact in the study we reviewed in the preceding chapter.[49]

However, during antenatal education it is emphasised across the board that the first hour is paramount to a good start. Missing the critical or sensitive hour, for very valid reasons, often causes mothers undue stress and disappointment. Many feel that they have failed before they have started.

Furthermore, human mothers don't always fall in love with their babies at first sight. Even a mother who has had an easy natural birth, with no intervention, may gaze at her newborn and be immediately reminded of Uncle George whom she never liked. She may therefore have difficulty bonding and breastfeeding during that first hour. Or worse, maybe Uncle George is in her room wanting to be the first to greet the baby!

In either case, it may be impossible for her to achieve those two tasks: bonding and breastfeeding, predetermined by experts as critical to growth and development during that first window of time. Instead, there will likely be some tension that may cause distress. Tension, stress, anxiety, fear, and embarrassment are feelings that reduce oxytocin pulsatility, often having negative consequences for breastfeeding.[50]

Of course, early close mother–baby body contact should be promoted, but in counterbalance, my clinical experience and research projects suggest that we don't have to be in such a hurry. We don't have to ensure all mothers initiate a "successful breastfeed" within an hour of birth in the delivery suite nor do we need to create anxiety for mothers who are separated for short periods from their babies. Skin-to-skin research findings support my clinical experience.

Bystrova and her colleagues clearly show that a full range of *labour ward* routines does not adversely affect any early feeding outcomes, including rates of exclusive breastfeeding.[51] However, Bystrova and her colleagues found that routines on the *postnatal ward* do.

Importantly, when on the postnatal ward, when mothers are proactive, keeping their sleeping babies at the right address during the first 48 hours, there are endless opportunities to initiate their breastfeeding relationship. Biological nurturing offers simple and easy ways to address latching problems, engorgement, sore nipples, sleepy babies, and low blood sugars before resorting to hand expression.[52,53]

People often ask me: "What do you mean? What are these easy ways?" A BN strategy that works a treat when any baby fights the breast is to encourage the mother to hand express directly into the baby's mouth while the baby, in a BN position, is latched but asleep on the breast. While mum occasionally expresses, drips and drops of colostrum build up in the baby's mouth. A mouthful of colostrum releases a swallow. A swallow often promotes a suck and a suck releases more milk. This slow cycle of active suckling is crucial for baby's learning. It is important for the baby to have a sense of mouth fullness, both from the breast and from the milk. The earlier the baby has experienced this sense of mouth fullness as a stimulus to swallow, the quicker the breastfeeding reflexes will be conditioned. Importantly, sleeping babies latch on and feed in biological nurturing positions and we discuss these mechanisms in depth in Chapter 14.

The biological nurturing perspective, therefore, refutes the discontinuous notion that the first hour is absolutely crucial to breastfeeding success. Plasticity, a term often used by neurologists to describe how people's brains become hardwired, underpins BN theory. Plasticity describes the incredible human capacity for adaptive change in response to a positive or negative environment. In other words, life experiences can continuously mould and enhance learning, growth, and development.

My 45 years of clinical practice suggest that there's not one critical window of time during which mothers must establish crucial competencies and achieve developmental milestones. Mothers and babies learn best within "their species-specific developmental habitats." For breastfeeding the habitat is "the mother's body, and her lactational apparatus".[54] Recreating the learning environment, which is "inseparable from a behaving body," often rescues any initial learning deficit.

What About the Preterm Baby?

The UK BFI standard provides excellent guidance about the preterm infant's needs. Certainly, the time to teach and encourage early manual expression is when sick or preterm babies are transferred to intensive care and separation will be prolonged. That really is a gift! Likewise, Morton's lovely video clips should be shown in all neonatal special care units. However, as soon as mother and baby are reunited, mothers can BN their sleeping babies at the right address, encouraging them to latch and actively suckle, as discussed above.

Many late preterm babies are able to breastfeed exclusively. Some, of course, will require supplements of expressed colostrum or a mix of mother's colostrum and artificial milk drink.[55] But it is time to stop extrapolating a good thing that works for a minority, vulnerable group of babies to all healthy term babies.

When Do Mothers Get Their Milk?

This is a question that many mothers ask. Professional response usually differentiates distinct stages of lactogenesis underpinned by discontinuity. Perceptions of milk insufficiency are the single most frequent reason mothers stop breastfeeding during the first two weeks. The fear that many mothers experience concerning milk insufficiency can be aggravated by well-intentioned but erroneous information they receive about how their milk will only "come in" on the third postnatal day. From a continuity perspective, this is incorrect as the milk "arrived" during pregnancy.[56]

On or around the third postnatal day, it's only the milk volume that increases to meet the baby's increasing needs. Initially, babies only ingest small, frequent amounts of colostrum, the first milk.[57] It is an advantage that there is not a copious milk supply in the first days as these frequent but short feeds help the baby locate the breast, learn how to latch, and coordinate sucking and swallowing with breathing.

Early breastfeeding patterns frequently differ from those established later, both in type, frequency and duration, often changing on a daily basis. For example, there is no uniformity even during the first 24 hours. Babies left in the cot may not cue or wake for a feed for six to eight hours. With each passing hour, tension can mount. Mothers wonder: "Why doesn't he wake up?"

In contrast, babies in BN, at the right address, may latch on and suck often, but the length of each episode may be very short and swallowing occasional. The first day patterns are often followed by periods of constant active feeding during the second and third postnatal days, suggesting that arbitrary demand-feeding schedules are inappropriate.[58] This "feeding frenzy" coincides with the time when many mothers fear they haven't got enough milk. Because the baby's drinking it all, their breasts can feel soft and empty. Biologically, this fear appears to be unsubstantiated as research findings suggest that the mechanisms for mother's breastmilk production are fully developed by around 20 weeks,[59] and many mothers release small quantities of milk during pregnancy.[60]

Mothers who miscarry often, regrettably, have copious milk production.[61] However, high concentrations of estrogen and other pregnancy-maintaining hormones inhibit milk release.[62]

We have known for many years that early active suckling and breast emptying promote high concentrations of prolactin, the milk-producing hormone.[63] In contrast, the release of oxytocin can be stimulated by merely thinking about the baby, with a mean peak in pulsatility at two and a half minutes. Except in the period immediately following birth, prolactin is only stimulated through mother/baby suckling, cheek-to-breast contact, non-nutritive sucking, and active milk transfer resulting in breast emptying.

Prolactin levels peak at 35–40 minutes from the start of a breastfeed.[64,65] These research findings indicate that practising BN during the first 48–72 hours, with lots of breast emptying, will help to regulate maternal milk supply earlier.

During the time of transitioning from womb feeding to mammary feeding, mothers may feel that they cannot put the baby down as one feed often blends into another. Babies often cry when mothers put them down. Mothers think that the baby is unsettled, which leads to misconceptions of an insufficient milk supply. In fact, babies usually cry when you put them down because their deep sleep function is immature. They awaken to find that they are no longer at the right address. We discuss neonatal behavioural state in depth in Chapter 14. Few babies cry when mums practise BN. The biological argument suggests that during at least the first three postnatal days – the time of metabolic adaptation – it is *not* normal to put the baby down for long periods of time.

How to Know That Baby Is Getting Enough

If you were to ask ten paediatricians how they know that the baby is getting enough milk, it is likely they would all say: "Weight gain." Many paediatricians believe that the baby should gain 15 to 30 grams each day.[66] If you asked ten lactation consultants the same question, they would probably say: "Correct attachment ensures effective feeding".[67] This agreement among groups of health professionals means that their assessments are "reliable" – here, reliable means that two or more health professionals evaluating the same mother–baby dyad obtain the same result. However, in the first 24 hours, healthy term babies often lose a variable percentage of their birthweight.

Research findings suggest that babies, on average, only ingest ≈7 ml per feed during the first 48 hours.[68] These facts invalidate daily weight as an indicator of adequate milk transfer. Validity means that the observations actually represent what they claim to measure. This definition challenges the trustworthiness of daily weights and other variables, such as the "correct latch," "leading in with the chin," or being "settled" after a feed as valid indicators of milk transfer. When professional assessments include invalid indicators of milk transfer, it can inadvertently make mothers worry.

Daily weight is a prime example. Consecutive infant feeding surveys reveal that concerns about milk insufficiency lead to unnecessary supplementation and early unintended breastfeeding cessation.[69-75] This often causes mothers to feel anxious, guilty, and disappointed. It sometimes triggers postnatal depression.[76] Indeed, focus groups in 2012 indicated that mothers worry about their milk production even when their baby is gaining normally.

The researchers concluded that our professional assessment and interaction with mothers can have unintended consequences, actually augmenting maternal anxiety.[77] Anxiety is strongly associated with low oxytocin pulsatility and reduced prolactin levels.[78] Taken together, these findings present a strong argument suggesting that one of our priorities is to reduce maternal anxiety.

Does That Mean That We Should Never Weigh Babies?

No, normally we weigh healthy term babies at birth, sometimes at hospital discharge, and at around two weeks when we would expect a baby to have regained her birthweight. Thereafter, monthly weights are all that is usually needed to indicate normal growth curves. However, healthy preterm babies should be weighed daily, also weigh any term baby for whom you have concerns or if your visual assessment suggests that there is excessive weight loss.

The Quest for the Correct Latch

The correct latch is the Holy Grail of breastfeeding, and many mothers fret and worry about achieving this. Yet the BN research data suggest that there's not one effective latch. The correct latch is the one that works, and this often varies from baby to baby. For example, the BN latch can be both superficial and pain-free, supporting effective milk transfer. This is because the BN latch is strongly associated with the neonate's degree of flexion or extension. The foetal attitude or the degree of flexion/extension prepares the way in which the newborn baby approaches the breast: leading in with the chin or with a trigeminal or full-facial head bob. Neonatal lie and attitude enrich breastfeeding observations and are subjects we discuss in great detail in Chapter 11.

The Myth of "Being Settled After A Feed"

We must remember that the baby has been held in the womb for nine months. Most babies appear settled after a feed when they are in mother's arms or on her body but as soon as baby is placed in a cot or cradle, he awakens. When this happens, instead of understanding that continuity of normal "habitat" has been disturbed, mothers often think that they haven't got enough milk and that is why the baby is not settled.

Health professionals believe that being "settled" and sleeping after a feed is an indicator of good milk transfer and satiety. Yet to my knowledge, there is no research data supporting this argument. Indeed, it sometimes works the opposite way: the "good baby" who spends hours asleep in the cot may fail to thrive. If latching reflex behaviours are released by positional interactions, as my data strongly suggest, then being settled in a cot is not a part of the equation.

Therefore, during the first six to eight weeks, being settled and sleeping soundly in a Moses basket or cot are not valid feed-by-feed indicators of milk supply, milk transfer, satiety, or neonatal well-being. Writing these into policy is just one more way that our cherished beliefs make mothers worry that their milk supply is insufficient. The BN perspective suggests that it is not normal for anyone to feel "settled" when arriving in a new place, let alone a newborn baby whose every system is immature.

Right after birth, being settled is not the aim. The aim is to make a successful transition from foetus to neonate. During the early weeks, babies who cry when placed in the cot after a feed are cueing. The baby usually stops crying as soon mum picks him up. The crying cues, therefore, only mean that the newborn baby was not at the right address. Babies often latch and feed again (despite having fed for X number of hours prior to being placed in the cot). This happens because that's what babies do at the right address; breastfeeding is their niche, their occupation. In that instance it does not necessarily mean that they are hungry or that mum has not got enough milk.

A final factor that often makes mothers uneasy is that they can't see how much milk is in their breasts. There are many valid ways to assess daily milk transfer without actually witnessing milk removal, without weighing the baby, and without assessing the latch.

As said previously, healthy term babies enter the world well fed with reserves that last approximately 48 hours. It's not the amount of milk ingested during the first postnatal hour that is important but rather the mutual awakening of the senses – vision, touch, audition, taste, smell, as well as thermoception, proprioception or body awareness, balance, and gravity. Of these, gazing, and especially the protogaze – or the first-time mother and baby look into each other's eyes – appears to release instinctual breastfeeding.[79]

What can be confusing is that there's a relatively small amount of colostrum compared to the prefilled bottles of artificial milk drink that you often see in hospital. We have emphasised that an initial small quantity of colostrum is actually beneficial. It's a laxative and it helps the baby to organise sucking with swallowing and breathing. The baby normally increases the mother's milk volume during the first 48 hours by suckling with good breast emptying. Initially, the baby sucks in succession several times, followed by a swallow. As the milk volume increases, and typically on the second or third day, there will be a 1:1 suck/swallow ratio with numerous sucking bursts.[80]

What goes in must come out and nappy assessments are essential. Each day, baby passes urine and the number of times corresponds to his age during the first week. That is, the first day, baby has at least one wet nappy, the second day, two and so on until day six or seven. Baby's urine is normally pale yellow and does not smell concentrated.

From then on, six to seven increasingly wet nappies over 24 hours are vital. During the first week, the baby's stool changes colour from black to brown, sometimes greenish to yellow (mustard colour). The colour changes always progress forward. In other words, yellow poo does not normally return to a brownish colour. The National Childbirth Trust has a very effective leaflet called *What's in a Nappy?* that informs mothers about infant stool changes.

As mum's milk volume increases, baby will have an increasing number of those suckling bursts in a relatively short period of time. For example, mum will hear her baby swallow maybe ten times successively in a 1:1 suck/swallow ratio. She will also see the jaw and ear move. Together with output, these are the most important daily indicators. But there are others. For example, babies who are drinking enough milk have a moist mouth after the feed. In the first weeks, mothers usually notice that their breast is smaller or softer after the feed. They are often thirsty. They may experience time appropriate womb contractions during a breastfeed. Importantly, both mother and baby have good muscle tone and look and act clinically well.

In the last two chapters, we have examined both continuous and discontinuous patterns in relation to how mothers and babies develop their innate capacity to breastfeed. These are observations developed, for the most part, after I finished my master's research. Knowledge is power, and I always share this information with mothers as it is invaluable in helping them transition into motherhood. However, at the time (circa 2001), what was important for me was to carry out research to test some of these theories.

CHAPTER 7

Exploratory and Descriptive Research

The Background Studies of Biological Nurturing

In 1997, Jane Hawdon, the pioneering metabolic researcher whose work influenced my practice, advertised for a research midwife. In a bi-centre randomised controlled trial, Hawdon and Williams, another leading consultant neonatologist, were examining the effects of supplementation upon breastfeeding and metabolic adaptation for healthy but moderately preterm infants.

Hawdon and DeRooy, one of her senior medical registrars, were also carrying out similar metabolic profiles for healthy but small and large for gestational age term babies. Supplementation was, prior to this research, routinely prescribed for these healthy, but vulnerable, babies considered at risk of hypoglycaemia. I jumped at the opportunity to work under their guidance and was seconded to the new position.

Having had clinical, albeit anecdotal, experiences of supporting exclusive breastfeeding for mothers whose babies were vulnerable but otherwise healthy, it was exciting to have close clinical supervision from experts like Hawdon, DeRooy, and Meek, another senior medical registrar. Their supervision sharpened and enhanced my clinical assessment skills. The concepts of suckling ketosis and counterregulation came to life.

An Exploratory Pilot Study

A feeding diary had originally been part of the research protocols but had been abandoned because no one could be bothered to complete it. Everyone just used the feed charts. Hawdon agreed that the mother/baby suckling diary could be used in addition to the feed charts. During the nine months of the secondment, I recruited over 50 mothers to the metabolic trial and piloted the suckling diary with 12 of them to explore biological nurturing (termed biological suckling at the time) as a strategy for a subset of mothers recruited for the metabolic studies who wanted to breastfeed exclusively.

Using a qualitative methodological approach, the aims were first to articulate biological nurturing as an intervention and second to examine if, and how, BN affected breastfeeding initiation. The suckling diary was the main data collection instrument. The metabolic research protocols were flexible, and when babies were breathing air, appeared healthy and infection free, I supervised their care on the postnatal ward.

I officially studied 11 healthy but moderately preterm babies (between 34 and 36 completed gestational weeks) and one healthy but small-for-gestational-age term baby. All were breastfed from birth. A key finding was that many healthy but moderately preterm infants can breastfeed exclusively from birth. Clinical midwifery and breastfeeding assessment skills, reflecting an understanding of metabolic adaptation, were crucial to avoid unnecessary supplementation.

Full results of the pilot study, undertaken for a MSc in midwifery,* are published elsewhere.[1] However, reviewing certain temporal findings, or spontaneous mother-specific breastfeeding styles, can help clarify the background concepts behind biological nurturing.

Temporal Findings

Biological nurturing measures temporal variables of two behavioural types: body/breast contact and active milk transfer. Through analysis of the diaries, I was able to calculate simple statistics for such proximate variables as suckling frequency, duration, and interval duration defined by Quandt[2] as key biological factors that impacted breastfeeding initiation. For example, for three of the mothers who spontaneously held their babies at birth, the mean holding time was one hour, ranging from 45 to 90 minutes.

This replicated other findings,[3] adding to an increasing body of evidence suggesting that the first hour following birth would be best spent greeting the baby. Interestingly, those mothers did not hold their babies in skin-to-skin contact. At the time of this study (1998), it was not yet standard practice for all mothers to hold their babies in this way.

---

* The MSc dissertation was awarded a distinction in June 2000, and a bound copy is available for consultation at London South Bank University Library.

The First 24 Hours

One of the first variables I examined was the number of BN episodes that occurred in the first 24 hours. An example of what we coded as a BN episode included the time the mother spent holding the baby in positions where the baby had unrestricted access to the breast versus the time the baby actually spent actively feeding. Active feeding was defined as sucking bursts with visible and/or age-specific audible swallowing.

The number of BN episodes varied quite a bit, ranging from 7 to 18, with a mean of 12. The neonates had unrestricted breast contact for a mean total of 7 hours and 40 minutes. However, there was a broad range in the breast contact time, with three mothers holding their babies in unrestricted breast access for approximately four hours and one mother for 16 hours. During the first 24 hours, babies actively breastfed, with vigorous sucking action, for a mean total of 2 hours and 35 minutes.

Those contact and active feeding times were longer than the time parameters in the new hypoglycaemia feeding guidelines that the midwives used on the ward.[4] In the guidelines, mothers were not encouraged to hold their babies outside of active feeding. The midwives therefore advised mothers to gently arouse sleeping babies after 8 or 12 postnatal hours if they had not yet awakened for a feed.

Mothers often ask questions about the length of time they should hold or feed their babies. The range of those findings was so wide, corresponding to individual needs, that it was difficult to give any fixed guidance. This is the reason why uniform temporal suggestions are absent from the "how to do it" part of biological nurturing.

The above findings, with the wide range of times, suggest that mothers should not be given specific numbers about how long they should hold or feed their babies. Just as the definition of neonatal hypoglycaemia is not a numbers game,[5] frequency of body contact and active milk transfer cannot be numbered, although sometimes it is helpful to give a time range rather than a specific number. Suggesting, for example, that mothers hold their babies "a lot," maybe a third of the day, works well for many.

One way to respond to mothers' temporal questions is to ask how long they *want* to hold the baby and then agree with their response if it is within those research parameters. Tell her that the evidence suggests that the number she gives is spot on accurate. Another way to respond to mothers' questions about how long they should hold their babies during the first 24 hours is to remind them that this time yesterday they were feeding the baby constantly. They couldn't put him down. This often makes mothers laugh. Laughter is such an important part of parenting, often clarifying the common sense responses.

Attending midwives and doctors also need indications of normal parameters to inform assessments. Without generalising, these statistics did just that, helping to frame temporal and frequency issues in a non-prescriptive way.

At the time, I was unaware of the central role played by the mother's posture. Nevertheless, during episodes of BN, I observed and described ten primitive neonatal reflex like movements appearing to stimulate feeding behaviours for the healthy, but vulnerable, babies studied. The presence or absence of the baby reflexes helped to determine clinical management as well as breastfeeding support.

Even if a baby reflex movement was only weakly present, I found it could release a cascade of innate baby-feeding behaviours. Seven of the 12 at risk babies that I studied required no supplementation with artificial milk drink from birth. The mean age at hospital discharge was six days and all 12 infants were exclusively breastfed at that time. At 4 postnatal months, 11 of the 12 infants were still breastfed (10 exclusively). Study numbers were too small to enable comparisons. However, these results were particularly encouraging when viewed alongside the UK national statistics. My findings on exclusive breastfeeding were unusual at the time for any healthy baby, let alone healthy but moderately preterm or small for gestational age babies.

Although the diary was particularly helpful for first time mothers, others found it a bit of a chore and only completed it because it was part of the research protocol. At the same time, I was developing an increased awareness of the role of the reflexes. I, therefore, attributed the achievement of these high rates of exclusive breastfeeding to the systematic release of the baby reflexes in BN positions, not the diary. The increase in breastfeeding duration across the small number of mother–baby pairs studied suggested that further research looking at biological nurturing was warranted.[6,7]

The PhD Study of Biological Nurturing

This previous work highlighted that keeping mothers' and babies' bodies together had a positive impact on breastfeeding, leading me to investigate what I now term biological nurturing. During the background studies, the how-tos of BN were more or less defined, identifying what looked like ten primitive neonatal reflexes that stimulated breastfeeding. However, if BN was to become a valid and reliable breastfeeding intervention, we needed further research to clarify the concepts and understand the underlying mechanisms.

Selecting a Research Design

All the mothers in the pilot study of BN were breastfeeding at six weeks. It was therefore tempting to pilot a randomised controlled trial (RCT), hypothesising that biological nurturing releases primitive neonatal reflexes (PNRs) and increases breastfeeding duration. A trial would allow me to compare two groups: BN as the experimental group and a positioning and attachment skills teaching group as the control. However, a hypothesis implies that the theory supporting the intervention is well developed and that the components are fully identified and defined operationally.[8] Following the pilot study, neither of these criteria was fully met.

As discussed in previous chapters, the concept of biological nurturing is purposefully abstract. A literature search revealed that many researchers have studied rooting and sucking, but few have looked at the role other PNRs might play in human feeding. Stepping and crawling, as well as tongue movements, hand-to-mouth, and hand massage have only been identified in breastfeeding studies carried out in skin-to-skin contact.

In those existing studies, most of the researchers focused on neonatal, but not maternal, competence. The mothers studied were specifically directed not to touch their babies as part of the protocol. This design allowed researchers to demonstrate neonatal competence, suggesting that babies have an innate capacity to breastfeed, even without the mothers' assistance.

However, this design had some serious limitations in that it did not include mothers and did not examine reciprocity or the critical interaction between the mothers' and babies' innate abilities. Furthermore, the behaviours that were observed were attributed to the effects of skin-to-skin contact, not the mothers' and babies' positions, nor the impact of neonatal behavioural states. Paediatricians identified positions and behavioural states as the key variables releasing PNR activity.[9-13] My prior qualitative study results concurred, identifying those two variables – positions and states – as related to the presence or absence of PNRs.

Another reason to carry out descriptive, rather than experimental, research concerns a thornier issue. The UK Medical Research Council highlights that descriptive studies supporting theoretical clarity are often omitted during the development of health interventions due to time and financial constraints. Many of the current protocols for assisting mothers to breastfeed were developed without proper evaluation and gold standard evidence to support their effectiveness. We now know, and our low rates of breastfeeding continuance support this, that many of these techniques and procedures do not work.

In the development of biological nurturing, it made scientific sense to try to avoid the same pitfalls. That is why I went back to the drawing board, selecting a descriptive-comparative design and a mixed-methods approach, enabling the systematic and objective identification of the different components of BN and how they interrelate. Nevertheless, it was also important to measure breastfeeding rates at both 2 and 6 weeks: not to find out cause and effect determinants, but to inform decisions about the feasibility of developing BN further as an intervention to support breastfeeding initiation. If the results showed that an equal number (or fewer) mothers were breastfeeding at these times than the UK national averages, then regardless of the findings for the mechanisms, the development of BN would be abandoned.

The immediate purpose of the PhD investigation, therefore, was not to test the effects of the BN intervention. Rather, it was to uncover the mechanisms of biological nurturing, establishing whether BN releases primitive neonatal reflexes as breastfeeding stimulants, as it appeared to do in my previous research. In addition, it was important to explore the overall contribution PNRs might make to infant feeding and to compare descriptions of any PNRs observed that appeared to stimulate feeding, in both the bottle and breastfeeding contexts.

When people undertake PhD research, there is a supervisory panel, and sometimes expert advisors, helping to maintain a high academic standard. For my study, both academic and clinical experts supported the work. The supervisory panel comprised a chairperson, two academic supervisors, and a clinical supervisor. A sub-group of breastfeeding experts was comprised of an International Board Certified Lactation Consultant and National Childbirth Trust breastfeeding counsellor, a La Leche League peer supporter, a cranial osteopath, and a consultant neonatologist.

A descriptive comparative study design was selected, using a mixed methods approach with videotaped observations as the primary method of data collection. One session was filmed either in hospital or at home, for both breast and bottle feeding mothers. In this book, we concentrate primarily on the findings for the breastfeeding group. A full description of the research design can be found in the thesis[*] and in a subsequent research article. [14] However, the specific research questions and outcome measures are displayed in Table 1. This brief description of the objectives can help you understand the results.

---

[*]   The PhD thesis won the inaugural Royal College of Nursing Akinsanya award in 2006, and a bound copy is available for consultation in the Royal College of Nursing Library Steinberg Collection. A PDF can be ordered from The British Library.

Table 1: Research Questions and Outcome Measures

Research Question	Outcome Measure
Can the components of BN be described? How do they interrelate and interact?	The description of the BN components and explanations for how they interact.
Does BN release PNRs? If so, how is BN influenced by the two key neurological variables: positions and states?	The identification and description of a number of PNRs as feeding stimulants across breastfeeding positions and neonatal behavioural states.
Can any PNRs be observed systematically to play a role in the feeding context?	Description of role, type and potential function.
Should BN be developed further as an intervention to support breastfeeding?	Breastfeeding duration at 2 and 6 postnatal weeks.

What About Skin-To-Skin Contact?

On the surface, babies whose mothers practise BN exhibit behaviours that are similar to those found in skin-to-skin contact.[15-17] Skin-to-skin contact is the positioning of the naked or nappy-clad infant near the naked mother's breast, on her chest, or between her breasts. Kangaroo care is a method originally designed for grossly preterm infants where mothers keep their babies in skin-to-skin contact. Like an incubator, the naked contact maintains baby's temperature while offering unrestricted access to the breast.[18] The breast crawl is a form of skin-to-skin contact often used immediately following birth: the mother is placed flat or semi-flat on her back and the baby lies prone on mum's chest.

In 1998, I was a fervent promoter of skin-to-skin contact for all the mothers in my preterm study. However, midwives on the labour ward preferred incubators and mothers on the postnatal ward often emphatically said that they did not want to undress. Many felt uncomfortable and/or worried that their babies would catch cold. Others experienced embarrassment at the very thought of being naked when greeting their friends and family.

RCTs demonstrate a striking thermoregulatory benefit associated with skin-to-skin contact. However, close physical BN contact in a state of light dress appeared to safeguard the neutral thermal environment necessary to reduce cold stress for the preterm infant. No mother in my study practised skin-to-skin contact, yet all of the preterm babies under my charge maintained normal temperature while lightly dressed. I became convinced that mothers know best and stopped insisting on skin-to-skin contact. As stated previously, at hospital discharge all were exclusively breastfeeding. At four months, 92% were breastfeeding exclusively. One mother was mixed-feeding.

Concurrently in Australia, Roberts and her colleagues were investigating whether differences in the outcomes for kangaroo care (KC) could be attributed to naked contact alone. Their study compared two groups of similar mother/moderately preterm infant dyads. Both groups of mothers cuddled their babies while sitting in rocking chairs. The KC group had skin-to-skin contact, while the standard care, conventional cuddling group had contact through normal clothing. Conventional cuddling produced outcomes equivalent to those of skin-to-skin contact (weight gain, temperatures, length of stay in the hospital, breastfeeding, Parental Stress Scale, and Parental Expectations Survey). The researchers concluded that conventional cuddling provides an equivalent alternative for mothers who do not feel comfortable with naked skin-to-skin contact.[19]

Three years later, Anderson and colleagues assessed what type of early contact mothers would choose and how long it would last during the first 48 hours. Similar mother–moderately preterm infant dyads were randomly assigned to an experimental group: a) where mothers could experience KC whenever they chose or a control group, b) where mothers could hold their infants wrapped in blankets whenever they chose. Skin-to-skin contact started at birth for the KC dyads. Upon transfer to the postnatal ward, the researchers strongly urged them to practise skin-to-skin contact as often as possible whereas, apparently, the control group received no guidance concerning frequency of baby holding. A follow-up study evaluating breastfeeding duration revealed that the KC dyads breastfed significantly longer than the controls.[20,21]

Currently, skin-to-skin contact is the gold standard of breastfeeding initiation and researchers seek to support their hypotheses by illustrating a plethora of benefits. Accordingly, Anderson et al. anticipated a high uptake of skin-to-skin contact. However, they encountered three surprise findings. First, following postnatal transfer, few KC mothers chose to practise skin-to-skin contact, despite enthusiastic daily encouragement from the researchers. The reasons given were very similar to those in my study – the arrival of visitors or staff preventing or interrupting skin-to-skin contact sessions, modesty, and a desire to be presentable and/or attractively dressed.

Second, KC mothers often preferred to hold their infants wrapped in blankets, explaining that they couldn't see their babies' faces and eyes in skin-to-skin contact. Although Anderson et al. cited the potency of the "en face gaze" first described by Klaus and Kennel in 1976, they failed to state that mothers were lightly dressed during that study.[22] Instead, they remained focused on skin-to-skin contact as the key variable. My research and Roberts' studies suggest that a thin layer of clothing between mother and baby doesn't interfere with bonding or breastfeeding.

Finally, Anderson et al. combined the time KC babies spent in wrapped holding with the time they spent in skin-to-skin contact. That overall total contact time was virtually double that of the controls, leading the researchers to conclude that birth skin-to-skin contact had increased the KC mothers' desire to hold their infants in blankets.

Their conclusion subtly shifts the focus of their study, disregarding the stated aim: maternal choices during early contact. However, it would have been valid if the researchers had checked with the mothers. As it stands, it's quite possible that the KC mothers only practised skin-to-skin contact to please the researchers.

Mothers of preterm infants are often as vulnerable as their babies, sometimes too frightened to even pick them up. The researchers discussed safe skin-to-skin contact practices, self-regulatory feeding, and taught mothers to recognise and value subtle infant feeding cues, constantly urging them to practise skin-to-skin contact. This was a clear bias. The control mothers did not receive this quality of attention. They were not given any guidance concerning safe wrapped holding or taught how best to hold their wrapped infants. Importantly, they were not constantly reminded to hold them. If they had been, it's likely that the percentage time of wrapped holding in the control group would have been significantly higher. If so, they probably would have breastfed for longer.

There's a strong argument to suggest that the guidance given to the experimental mothers was more valuable than the skin-to-skin contact itself. In research language, this common bias is called the Hawthorne Effect. These serious limitations hinder the validity of their overall conclusion stating that skin-to-skin contact increases breastfeeding duration.[23]

Interestingly, Anderson and colleagues inadvertently demonstrate that both skin-to-skin contact and wrapped holding benefit breastfeeding, replicating both Roberts' and my findings. An alternative conclusion is that mothers should choose the form of early contact that best meets their needs and be encouraged to hold their babies frequently.

Versatility of Early Mother–Baby Contact

Skin-to-skin contact is one way to positively influence breastfeeding by keeping mothers and babies together, but it's not the only way. Arguably, dress state should always be a mother's choice. Choice, continuity and control were the three Cs of childbirth during the 1990s. Today, one can ask: is it not time to apply these principles to postpartum care?

Understanding Cause and Effect

Skin-to-skin contact, biological nurturing, eye-to-eye contact, wrapped holding, conventional cuddling, en face gazing, rooming-in, and babywearing. This incredible variety of early mother–baby contact makes it difficult to understand which variables lead to successful breastfeeding, in other words, which ones are the independent variables.

The BN doctoral research suggested that interactions between the mothers' and babies' bodies – not skin-to-skin contact – stimulated a range of what appeared to be inborn reflexes. Babies sleeping cheek to breast exhibited mouthing, licking, nuzzling, and nesting behaviours. Stepping and rooting movements, searching, and latching onto the breast occurred in sleep and awake states. Active sucking and swallowing were commonly followed by sleeping and then re-latching behaviours. Mothers, gazing at their babies and actively engaged, appeared to elicit these behaviours spontaneously without skin-to-skin contact. Maternal cues appeared to trigger babies' reflexes or baby cues released maternal response. Together these appeared to be the variables necessary for successful breastfeeding.[24]

Future Research

Biological nurturing research has not ended with the doctoral work exploring the mechanisms. As related in Chapter 4, Gadroy found a significant difference in breastfeeding duration following BN intervention on day two compared to controls. Further trials are needed with larger sample sizes.[25]

However, more research like Roberts' study is needed to focus specifically on maternal choice and type of early contact. For example, one could hypothesise that equivalent outcomes will be found when comparing biological nurturing contact with skin-to-skin contact and evaluating mothers' experiences.

The endpoint of research projects investigating biological nurturing needs to be a valid and reliable intervention that supports breastfeeding initiation – and ultimately, this is my aim. For biological nurturing, validity means that the BN intervention increases maternal enjoyment and breast-feeding duration. Reliability means that two or more practitioners using BN will support the same mother in a similar way, making the same assessment of milk transfer. To help achieve these endpoints, an RCT is underway in Italy (see Appendix).

In fact, the development of any health intervention is complex, which is why the Medical Research Council provides specific guidance in this area. The council defines a complex intervention as one where there are "various inter-connecting parts or components that interrelate and interact" to produce the desired effect. The challenge is to identify the "active ingredients" or those components that are essential to attain the expected outcome, i.e., the independent variable(s). The PhD study made an important contribution towards the achievement of that aim.

CHAPTER 8

Biological Nurturing: The Active Ingredients and Mechanisms

It is difficult to define biological nurturing in ways that capture the magic of the approach. During BN certification workshops, small groups of health professionals and mothers write how they would describe biological nurturing in simple terms. Some of these definitions are listed below.

Table 2: BN Breastfeeding Companions Define BN

Question: In a few sentences, define biological nurturing for a mother or a colleague
BN is a new breastfeeding approach based upon mother–baby interactions that optimise the spontaneous expression of innate behaviours, helping mothers welcome their babies, promoting bonding and nutrition. The BN approach places mothers at the centre; mothers are active agents, as competent as their babies. Mothers, not health professionals, are responsible for managing breastfeeding. *Martine, Speech Therapist, France*
BN has to do with a semi-reclined maternal position that opens her body to welcome her baby. This aids mother–baby interactions, emphasising continuity from womb to world. BN is based upon the natural, the physiological, maternal instincts, and baby reflexes. In BN, the nursing couple knows how to do it. Our role is to let them discover each other. *Jessica, Midwife, France*

Biological nurturing is an innovative approach to breastfeeding based on theories of continuity from womb to world. The term collectively designates a set of maternal postures and neonatal positions, maternal, and baby innate behaviours and states. *Alex, biologist, Italy*

Biological nurturing is a different approach to breastfeeding initiation. It has mother's comfort and self-assurance as a priority and is based on an interaction between babies' and mothers' positions, innate behaviours and states. In our practice this kind of early approach enhances breastfeeding duration. *Annamaria, Midwife, Italy*

BN is a new approach that normalises breastfeeding. It is focused on the mother and is based on a semi-reclined position that releases innate behaviours making things easier for both the mother and her newborn. *Simona, Paediatrician, Italy*

BN is not just a method of feeding, it introduces new ways to think about continuity from womb to world and aims to promote empowerment of mother–baby. *Francesca, Midwife, Italy*

BN is a bridge between nature and culture. It describes certain mother–baby postures and states that release the natural and instinctive behaviour in both mother and baby, which supports and enhances breastfeeding. *Marta, Midwife, Italy*

Biological nurturing is intuitive breastfeeding: it's a philosophy as well as an approach that prioritises mother–baby reciprocity. Mothers instinctually release their babies' innate behaviours…at the same time, the inborn neonatal competency awakens the mother's instincts. *Angélique, Nurse, Switzerland*

Biological nurturing follows on from fetal life, a protective approach that helps babies deal with the sudden onset of gravitational effects. Traditionally these have often thwarted the expression of archaic baby feeding reflexes present from 34 gestational weeks.
In optimising maternal comfort, BN gives breastfeeding back to mothers, suggesting that they are as competent as their babies. *Frédéric, Doctor in pharmacology at one of three breastfeeding-friendly pharmacies in France*

Importantly, biological nurturing is a multifaceted, holistic intervention. We can talk about components or ingredients, but to truly understand BN, you must recognise the synergistic relationship between them. The active ingredients – maternal postures, neonatal positions, and the positional subcomponents (neonatal lie and attitude within the positions and semi-ischial or sacral sitting within the postures) together with the mother's and baby's behavioural states – are always present, but, unexpectedly, these variables keep changing.

In BN, as in other complex systems, the total effect is truly greater than the sum of its individual parts. Moreover, mothers and babies are constantly adding another dimension, their personal touch, so the number of BN active ingredients varies. For example, some babies don't root. They just quickly zero in and latch. Unsurprisingly, their mothers usually don't try to latch them or help them latch. However, other babies take their time, licking, head bobbing or mouthing before latching, and their mothers often actively participate.

In other words, all mothers and babies do not exhibit all of the innate behaviours observed during each BN episode, nor do these behaviours always present in the same sequence. This is in sharp contrast to findings in skin-to-skin contact that we looked at in Chapter 5 where researchers detail a single behavioural sequence beginning with the birth cry and ending with grasping the nipple, suckling, and sleeping. As discussed, mothers were discouraged from helping, moving, or shifting their babies' positions.[1] In comparison, during BN episodes, the number and sequence of behaviours appears to be triggered by, and tailored to, either the baby's or the mother's immediate and constantly changing needs.

Knowledge of this human diversity has a tremendous influence upon how we support mothers. Biological nurturing support has to do with accompaniment. The mother is the expert. We remain in the background. Most mothers do not require help or instructions. If there are any problems, your support becomes more like solving a human jigsaw puzzle rather than teaching or showing mothers breastfeeding routines. The BN jigsaw pieces belong to everyone but how they're joined results in an individualised innate breastfeeding picture.

In the event of difficulties, first you observe how the BN components are already assembled. Then you quickly identify the active ingredients and how to piece them together in a more productive way based upon your observations of continuity from womb to world. One way to assemble the BN jigsaw is illustrated in Figure 9.

Figure 9: The Biological Nurturing Jigsaw

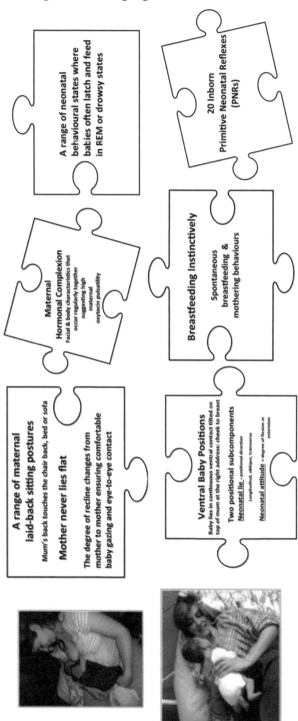

Figure 10 displays three photos of mothers and babies illustrating the diversity of BN practice. No matter what the position, two positional features remain constant: 1) maternal back, neck, and shoulder support, and 2) the close, constant ventral body-to-body contact as the babies' body curves are in close juxtaposition with the mothers' or with the environment.

In the photos on the left and lower right, the maternal body takes the full weight of the baby, whereas in the upper right picture, the baby's feet, calves, thighs, and part of the baby's abdomen are in close apposition with the bed.

The Mechanisms of Biological Nurturing

The Oxford dictionary defines a "mechanism" as "a system of mutually adapted parts working together … a means by which a particular effect is produced." Doctoral analysis revealed that laid-back sitting postures and neonatal close ventral/frontal positions are the primary components of the *BN system*. Those two parts are *"mutually adapted and working together"* to release instinctual breastfeeding behaviours for both mothers and babies even when babies were in sleep states.

Pressure from constant ventral contact releases movement, rippling to and fro from navel to limbs. Friction from the baby's limbs brushing against mum, together with gravity, keeping baby on top, are *the means* by which the *particular effect* or successful breastfeeding is *produced*. This is not surprising as the laid-back maternal sitting postures always use gravity positively, ensuring close constant tummy contact and making it possible for every part of the baby's front, but especially his thighs, calves, and feet tops, to brush up against a maternal body contour or against part of the environment.

There will always be a range of baby positions and mother postures whose interactions release instinctive breastfeeding behaviours for mothers and inborn baby reflexes as breastfeeding stimulants. This positional individuality promotes maternal comfort while she looks at her sleeping baby or gazes into her baby's eyes. This special mother–baby communication usually releases pain-free effective latching, leading to rhythmic suckling bursts and successful milk transfer. The range and variety in positions depends upon many factors, including positional continuity from womb to world, the degree of privacy, anthropometric characteristics, such as the height of the mother and the weight and maturity of the baby.

If you do not teach mothers "comfortable upright" or "side-lying positions," or "natural breastfeeding" positions, they often spontaneously use a degree of

Figure 10: As many variables as there are mothers

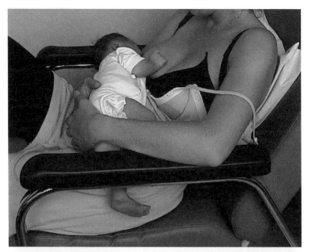

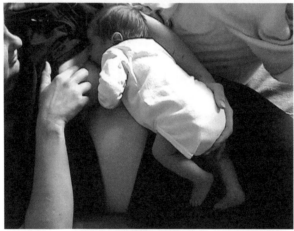

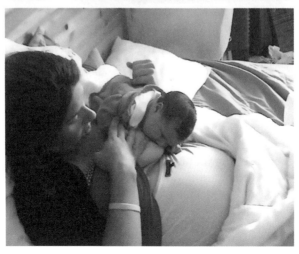

Figure 11: The Mechanisms of Biological Nurturing

Mothers – Laid-Back Sitting Postures
- Open the mother's body
- Increase her torso dimensions
- Make the body region between sternum & pubis available to her baby
- Optimise comfortable baby gazing & eye-to-eye contact

Gravity
- Pins baby to mother's body
- Reduces intensity & amplitude of PNRs
- Frees mother's hands to groom & stroke her baby

Babies – Ventral Positions
- Species-specific to quadrupeds
- No back, head, or neck pressure required
- Multidirectional approach to mum's breast
- Babies lie around the breast like the hands of a clock, instantly increasing the number of baby positions from 3 to 360
- Promote continuity in positional lie & attitude from womb to world
- Normalise longitudinal & oblique lies
- Close constant ventral contact smooths movement & releases PNRs enabling locomotion.
- Work with (not against) gravity.

Baby Gazing and Eye-To-Eye Contact
- Promote postnatal continuity of oxytocin from pregnancy & labour
- Increase maternal oxytocin pulsatility

High Oxytocin Pulsatility
- Releases mothers' breastfeeding instincts
- Promotes spontaneous mothering behaviours protecting baby's breathing, warmth, & sleep

Biological Nurturing is proactive. Mothers take the lead; they hold their sleeping babies during the early days
- Keeps baby at the right address
- Reduces crying
- Mothers get to know their babies sooner, boosting maternal confidence
- Reduces intensity & amplitude of PNR expression
- Promotes spontaneous latch in REM & drowsy sleep states
- Increases breastfeeding frequency mimicking womb feeding aiding metabolic adaptation
- Gives mothers time to sort latching difficulties or sore nipples
- REM states optimise brain development & early learning, therefore babies coordinate sucking with swallowing & breathing earlier.

body slope that meets their needs at the time. This, in turn, often enhances baby gazing and eye-to-eye contact, without placing strain on the mother's shoulders or neck. Contrary to traditional breastfeeding dogma, biological nurturing changes breastfeeding into a two-way relationship characterised by reciprocity. The BN mechanisms are summarised in Figure 11.

Importantly, of all the mechanisms, the positive use of gravity for a human baby, born a quadruped, is probably the most striking. This is because the baby's ventral positional needs contrast sharply with those of his upright bipedal mum who has a species-specific drive to be vertical. Biological nurturing helps to mediate this positional paradox and we discuss this further in Chapter 12.

Note what this breastfeeding counsellor from Birmingham describes:

◆

TESTIMONIAL

I notice that in BN the baby is most definitely "tummy to mummy" in all positions, as this is a fundamental part of releasing the reflexes to propel the baby toward the breast. I have seen this many times. In BN, the baby may be diagonal to the mother's body with bottom held by mother's hand, which falls naturally also in a diagonal position resting in her lap. A horizontal hold often seems rather uncomfortable. There appears to be a lot of research to support this BN view. I appreciate the mother's feeding position is different – being more laid back.

◆

In the next chapters we examine each BN component in depth and relate the important role gravity plays in greater detail. But as described earlier, mothers' and babies' bodies are biologically designed to work together to ensure the survival of the species. The real magic of BN occurs when you assess and support all the active ingredients working together.

CHAPTER 9

Primitive Neonatal Reflexes

Peope from many disciplines have shown a certain fascination with primitive neonatal reflexes (PNRs), from the early baby biographers, such as Darwin[1] and Preyer,[2] to physicians such as Peiper,[3] who catalogued more than 50 PNRs, making phylogenetic comparisons. Developmental psychologists, such as Piaget,[4] who was also a baby biographer, Illingworth,[5] and Gesell, Ilg, and Ames,[6] also introduced PNR assessments, using the work of well-known paediatricians.

Indeed, in-depth understanding about PNRs comes from five landmark medical assessment instruments that were developed in the 1960s and 1970s.[7-11] These medical assessments integrated many PNRs as components of the neurological evaluation of the newborn baby. For example, the Brazelton and Nugent *Neonatal Behavioural Assessment Scale*, now in its fourth edition, evaluates 18 PNRs, and is used by clinicians and researchers the world over.[12]

Primitive neonatal reflexes are sometimes called archaic reflexes. Both expressions are collective terminology representing three kinds of innate movement: inborn, unconditioned reflexes, spontaneous reactions, or innate responses to environmental or endogenous stimuli. Together with infant state and tone, PNRs are used to map gestational age and to assess neurological function. For example, the Moro reflex, one of the first PNRs researchers documented, is probably the best known among health professionals. Parents may be more familiar with the stepping reflex, where the examiner, holding the baby around the chest, brushes the soles of the baby's feet against a hard surface. This releases automatic walking movements.

PNRs are simple reflexes supported by an intact nervous system. The medical evaluation also serves as a screening test. The absence of an expected PNR, or the presence of one for longer than expected, are considered predictors of concurrent neuropathology.

Successful feeding also depends upon an intact nervous system and three PNRs: rooting, sucking, and swallowing were described formally as infant feeding stimulants in the paediatric neonatal assessment instruments. More recently, several researchers, examining the effects of skin-to-skin contact, have introduced a potential feeding role for other PNRs. For example, Righard and Frantz added hand-to-mouth, and stepping and walking interpretations in the *Delivery Self-Attachment* video.[13]

Widström named hand-to-mouth, stepping, and crawling reflexes, describing what she termed predictable behavioural patterns of how the baby held in skin-to-skin contact finds the breast during the first hour following birth.[14] These patterns were then illustrated in a video called *Breastfeeding: The Baby's Choice*.[15] This is now termed the breast crawl and is the form of birth skin-to-skin contact that we discussed in Chapter 5.[16,17]

In the preterm context, brushing techniques are central to the release of rooting. In the Newborn Individualized Developmental Care and Assessment Program (NIDCAP), developed by Als in the U.S. and Nyqvist in Sweden, "licking" is listed as a developmental observation in the Preterm Infant Breastfeeding Behaviour Scale (PIBBS).[18,19] Results from the background studies articulating biological nurturing suggested that there were many more PNRs that might play a role in breastfeeding initiation, and that skin-to-skin contact was not the independent variable or the principle releaser.

Schools of Thought on Neurological Assessment

Different schools of thought inform the neurological assessment of the term and preterm infant. Each school draws upon Prechtl's extraordinary work giving detailed description of the PNRs and their releasers.[20] However, there are four dominant and differing perspectives or neurological "world views" that underpin a philosophy of neonatal evaluation: *Le tonus*, or muscle-tone, paradigm developed by the French school[21] and the Dubowitz model in England,[22] the reflexological approach developed by the Dutch school;[23] the behavioural-driven assessment developed by the American school;[24] and a relatively new ontogenetic-adaptation paradigm, where general neonatal movements (GMs) are observed and interpreted as predictors of long-term neurological outcomes.[25]

PNRs are weakly present by 28 completed weeks of gestation, and the strength of PNR response is a major predictor of maturation. The Dubowitz model focuses, for the most part, upon prematurity, and the stick figures of babies in flexion and extension are recognised the world over.[26]

Gestational age, neonatal positions, and neonatal behavioural states are the variables that have been shown to influence both PNR strength of reaction or response and the qualitative expression (the simple presence or absence) of the PNRs. Equipped with this knowledge, Prechtl, in landmark work studying over 1,500 babies, standardised the evaluation techniques and scoring procedures used during the neonatal evaluation. Each reflex was described and the procedures and techniques for its release minutely detailed, and these were understandably inflexible. Reliability was paramount. Two examiners assessing the same baby would need to attain the same result, as the examination was designed to detect pathology versus well-being.

The assessment literally said, "yea or nay" to nervous-system function. Therefore, to achieve high interassessor reliability, Prechtl standardised everything, including the height of the examination table and the lighting and heating in the room. He defined neonatal behavioural states and those examination positions that would release optimal PNR responses. That is why most of the PNRs are released and assessed when the baby is in a quiet alert behavioural state, even though PNRs can often be observed in sleep states.[27]

The Impact of Neonatal Position

Paediatricians use three positions to release and assess the reflexes. They place the baby supine, prone, or in ventral suspension, where the examiner holds the baby around the thorax with feet dangling. Finger and plantar grasping, sucking, rooting, and the Babinski reflex, a kind of a toe-fanning response, are among those examined when babies are supine.

When babies lie prone, such spontaneous responses as bringing the head to the midline, head lifting and crawling are released. In ventral suspension, automatic stepping and placing are triggered. Placing is described as a lifting and placing movement in response to brushing the top of the baby's foot against a hard surface, usually the examination table. Figure 12 illustrates the placing response in ventral suspension.

What Do PNRs Have to Do with Breastfeeding?

People often wonder what such movements as placing, finger or plantar grasping, or a Babinski toe fan could possibly have to do with infant feeding. For the

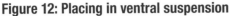

Figure 12: Placing in ventral suspension

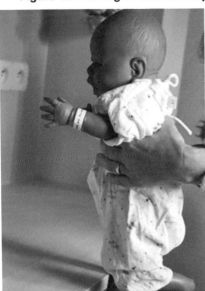
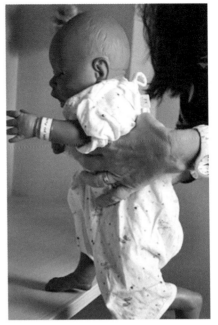

The examiner brushes the top of baby's foot against a hard surface.
The baby spontaneously lifts and places her foot on the hard surface.

answers to these questions, we need to look more closely at biological nurturing.

The overall purpose of my PhD study was to investigate primitive neonatal reflexes as the primary components of biological nurturing. Having observed PNR-like movements appearing to stimulate feeding during episodes of BN and because all healthy normal babies have these reflexes at birth, I thought that increased understanding of these inborn movements might yield further knowledge about how best to support breastfeeding initiation for healthy term babies.

Primitive Neonatal Reflexes: Number and Classification

In my study, 54 mother–baby pairs were videotaped and studied: 40 in the breastfeeding group and 14 in the bottle feeding group. Twenty PNRs were identified, described, compared, and validated in the feeding context with high (0.8) interrater agreement. PNRs were categorised into four types: endogenous, rhythmic, motor, and anti-gravity. Today five feeding functions can be suggested: releasing, cueing, searching or finding PNRs, sustaining or stabilising reflexes or those maintaining the baby in place, and the PNRs that promote milk transfer. The PNRs together with the type and function are displayed in Figure 13.

The Role Played by PNRs: Unexpected Findings

Jerky movements pushing the baby away from the breast, head shaking, leg scrambling, flinging, arm thrashing, boxing, fighting, scratching, and leg cycling movements that looked like kicking – we never anticipated such a description of PNRs in the feeding context. On the other hand, we sometimes observed the same movements as smooth and coordinated. In other words, the same reflexes looked like they could either help the baby find the breast, latch on, and sustain milk transfer, or they appeared to thwart latching and successful breastfeeding.

Researchers have always described the rooting and sucking reflexes as feeding stimulants. Therefore, this dual role that the PNRs appeared to play caught us by surprise. At the same time, during data analysis, the mother's breastfeeding position emerged as unquestionably the single most important variable, either releasing the reflexes as stimulants or as breastfeeding

Figure 13: Primitive Neonatal Reflexes: Type and Function

Reflex Outcomes: 20 PNRs Identified[28]	
Endogenous *(cues or releasing reflexes)* Hand to mouth, Mouth gape Tongue dart/lick Arm cycle, Leg cycle Finger flexion/extension Hand/foot flex	**Motor** *(searching/finding reflexes)* Palmar, plantar grasp Stepping, Crawling Placing Babinski
Rhythmic *(milk transfer or sustaining reflexes)* Suck Masseter (Jaw jerk) Swallow	**Anti-Gravity** *(searching/finding reflexes)* Head righting Head lifting Rooting Head bobbing

Described/compared, validated ► Inter-observer agreement 0.82

barriers. As a result, we needed to formulate research definitions to describe a range of maternal breastfeeding postures in a systematic and objective fashion. These definitions will be illustrated and discussed in Chapter 10, where we explore the postural causes of this dual role, explaining how an inborn reflex response like rooting, which is "normally" supposed to stimulate latch, could be transformed into a negative influence resulting in latch failure.

Latch Failure

Consecutive UK feeding surveys characterise latch failure either as "fighting the breast" or as "breast refusal," where a baby who should be hungry is either too sleepy to latch or fails to suck.[29-35] Objective descriptions of what is visible or audible, however, are sparse.

Gohil, an Indian paediatrician, offers a vivid description of what he calls a new breastfeeding behaviour observed during engorgement. Termed "breast boxing," he describes some PNR-like movements associated with latch failure that we often observed in my study.[36]

> It was observed that the infant does not suckle and pushes himself away with his fisted hands at the breasts or abdomen of the mother, and kicks away at the mother's abdomen and avoids feeding.[37]

My data suggested that these kicking and pushing away behaviours were often combined with increasingly frenetic activity and to and fro horizontal head shaking, thwarting latch. Typically, the baby was in a quiet alert state at the start of the feed, and after about a minute, if latch was not successful, side-to-side head rooting movements increased in frequency and intensity. These were often accompanied by the hand-to-mouth reflex, where the hungry baby appeared to prefer sucking on his fist instead of the breast.

At the time, the UK Baby Friendly Initiative[38] discussed these side-to-side head shaking movements in their training manual, suggesting that mothers often interpret these as the baby "saying no" to breastfeeding. See video clip 4 to view these common side-to-side head shaking movements.

At the first videotaped episode in my study, over half the breastfed babies displayed these negative behaviours, preventing them from latching. The UK BFI was quick to reassure that, contrary to maternal interpretation, this is "normal behaviour," and I agree with this point. However, when mothers sit upright the normal reflex expression often prevents latch.

Rooting can be characterised by a range of movement – the cardinal reflex (lip twitches), exaggerated side-to-side head shaking, the hand-to-mouth reflex, and arm and leg cycling are all an integral part of the "normal" behavioural rooting repertoire of the neonate. However, we observed systematically that, in certain positional situations, these inborn movements appear to be obstructive due to gravity. In certain positions, the force of gravity appeared to pull the mothers and babies apart and override the normal nature of the reflex response. We discuss gravitational mechanisms in depth in Chapter 13.

Video 3: Hand to mouth reflex thwarts latch

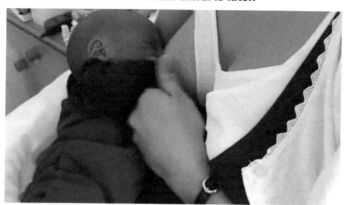

youtu.be/zX_7mQ0krfs

When mothers sit upright, babies often appear to prefer sucking on their fists rather than their mother's breast. In response, mothers often complain that they haven't got enough hands to breastfeed.

Video 4: Horizontal rooting reflex thwarts latch

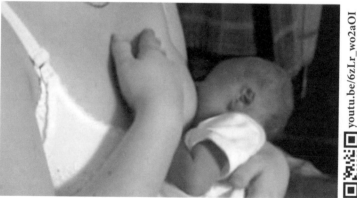

youtu.be/6zLr_wo2aOI

"Sometimes a newborn baby 'roots' for the breast. He moves his head from side to side as if he is saying 'no'. However, this is normal behaviour"[39]

How Does Position Affect the Role of the Reflexes?

Those mothers experiencing the negative PNR effects were either lying on their sides or sitting upright – bolt upright or leaning slightly forward – as they had been taught. Upright mothers often placed their babies on a pillow, lying transversely in front of and at right angles to their bodies, and although the baby was often "tummy to mummy," there was usually a gap or angle between the mother's and baby's bodies. The baby's thighs, calves, and feet were often in contact with thin air. Importantly, mothers *had to hold* their babies in positions where they applied pressure along the baby's back to keep him on the pillow and/or at breast level. I have termed this *dorsal feeding*.

In dorsal feeding, the more the mother struggled to elicit mouth gape, leading in with the chin, the tighter she gripped the baby's back. This firm grip often extended to the baby's neck or head. The firmer the grip, the more the baby struggled with frantic arm and/or leg cycles, increasing in strength and amplitude as the baby quickly worked himself up to a crying state.

Dorsal Feeding

Peiper, a German physician, whom many consider the founder of child neurology, compares positional phenomena across species and assumes that dorsal feeding (where mothers must physically hold their babies' backs) is uniquely human.[40] In fact, we have always believed that our babies, unlike some of our mammalian cousins, are obligate dorsal feeders (i.e., need to feed with pressure on their backs). Whether breast or bottle feeding, a baby who is an obligate dorsal feeder always needs back pressure to maintain positional stability and to keep the baby at breast level, regardless of whether the mother is sitting upright or lying on her side. You can see how human mothers need to hold their babies, applying this pressure down the baby's back in Figure 14.

Frontal Feeding

In contrast, my research on biological nurturing positions found that our human babies may breastfeed best when they are not in the traditional holds where mothers must apply back and/or neck pressure. As soon as mothers lie back, and only three mothers did this spontaneously in the first videotaped episode, their babies are immediately in what Peiper termed a full abdominal position. I refer to this as a frontal feeding position. In these full chest and tummy positions, another baby reflex was observed – a pendular or head bobbing movement, which appeared to be released from

Figure 14: Dorsal Breastfeeding Positions

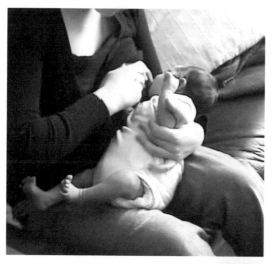

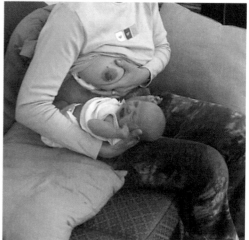

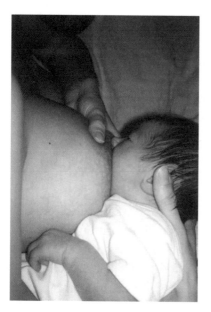

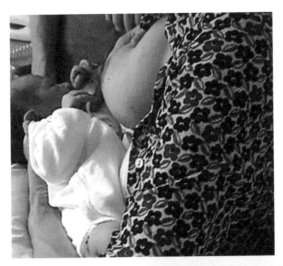

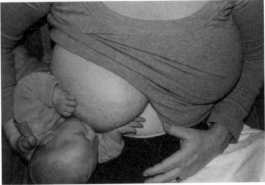

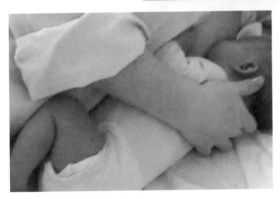

This figure illustrates dorsal feeding across the range of well known baby holding techniques: clutch or rugby/football hold, cradle and cross cradle hold, and side-lying.

Video 5: The woodpecker reflex thwarts latch

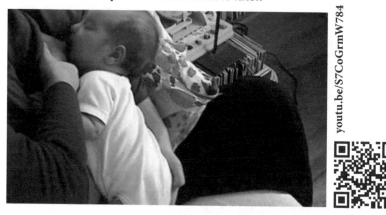

youtu.be/S7CoGrmW784

Do you see how the baby bobs his head like a little woodpecker? Unfortunately, the mother's upright posture maintains the baby in a vertical position. Notice baby's feet are unsupported. These factors contribute to latch failure.

Video 6: The woodpecker reflex aids latch

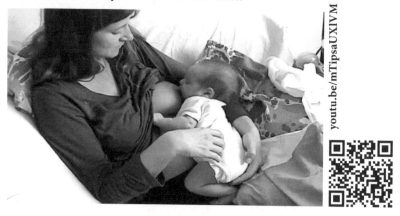

youtu.be/mTipsaUXIVM

Compare this video clip with the last one (number 5). Do you see how as the same mother increases her degree of recline, she opens her body. Her baby, reorients himself while she helps him latch. The change in degree of maternal recline initially disorients the baby but head bobbing (the woodpecker reflex) now aids latch, and mother and baby reciprocity ensures a quick and easy latch.

a fixed point in the baby's spine.

Peiper also documents this movement, previously observed by Prechtl, suggesting that vertical pendular movements stimulate latching in non human, abdominal feeding mammals. This includes animals such as puppies and hamsters, whose tummies hug the ground when they feed.[41]

I termed this position "frontal feeding" because observations suggested that it was not just the abdomen that was involved. You see in the video clip how the baby's entire torso, extending from sternum to pubis, is implicated. In full-frontal positions, the baby's thighs, calves, and feet tops are also spontaneously applied either to the mother's body or to a part of the environment – the bed, sofa, chair, bed clothes, etc.

Babies in frontal-feeding positions latched on more quickly and easily, and they also had some common points. First, their mothers were semi-reclined, but not all to the same degree of body slope. Second, the baby was neither held vertically nor parallel to the mother's body. Rather, he often positioned himself lying longitudinally (up and down) or obliquely on top of his mother. In other words, the baby always lay prone but, importantly, slanted with a natural physiological body tilt. This upward tilt was due to the gradient provided by the gentle maternal body slope.

The frontal feeding baby often approached the breast using the pendular head bobbing reflex, which most often involved the entire trigeminal area of the baby's face. Importantly, mothers did not have to hold the baby: no back, neck, or head pressure was required or necessary to achieve positional stability or to maintain the baby at breast level. Instead, gravitational forces helped to keep the baby on the mother's body. Gravity also appeared to make the reflexes smoother and more coordinated, aiding latch and sustaining milk transfer, as Nikki Lee, an American lactation consultant, describes.

◆

TESTIMONIAL

I have integrated [biological nurturing] into my 18-Hour Interdisciplinary Breastfeeding Management Course for the U.S. I show pictures from your article and discuss laid-back breastfeeding. I show the video clip about infant reflexes that can either help or hinder breastfeeding. Almost everyone can recognise the baby with the frantic arm and leg cycling and is very impressed with the change once the mother lies back. I shudder to remember how many babies whose legs and arms I held tightly so a mother could breastfeed... we learn and grow, thank goodness!!

Another thing; when I worked in labour and delivery and postpartum, I would see babies doing that "playing" at the breast. They would root and root and root and not latch on. I thought it was an impact of the epidural!! Thank you for your wonderful work.

◆

Andrea, a breastfeeding counsellor from the UK, described her personal experiences with her first baby, and how health professionals misunderstood the PNRs her baby was exhibiting.

◆

TESTIMONIAL

Suzanne, I just wanted to share my own experience with you. When my first daughter was born (nearly 8 years ago), I breastfed her in a sitting position (as been told and taught) but was never able to put her down afterwards without her waking and screaming. So we came to the agreement (me and her) that I would start feeding her in a nearly sitting up position and then gradually slouch back (till reaching BN position), which would leave us both happy. After a feed she would wriggle herself into a nice position and would sleep or just watch the world go by.

One day, just after such a feed the midwife came to see me. Jana (my daughter) lifted her head to see what was happening and the midwife said straight away "Don't let her do that, she will damage her neck."

A few weeks later I had my check up at the GP and Jana was screaming her head off when I lay down on the examination bench. So I said to the GP, I will just hold her while you get on with the examination (to the GP's dismay). I put Jana on my tummy (having propped myself up as much as I could) and she was lifting her head to see where she was. Again, the GP said "She will damage her neck if she lifts her head so high. Don't encourage it. You are spoiling her if you always hold her." I was in tears afterwards till I spoke to my own mother who simply smiled and said "That's what they told me as well. Just ignore it, go with your instincts and if any professionals challenge you, well, tell them what they want to hear, it makes your life easier, but in our family no one has let their babies cry and they all turned out well." I can't believe, that just 8 years ago they actively discouraged head bobbing etc.

◆

The common components of each approach are compared in Table 3.

Table 3: Upright and Side-lying vs. Biological Nurturing Postures

PNRs often released as barriers, thwarting latch or causing breast fighting	PNRs often released as stimulants, aiding easy and effective latch
Mother sits bolt upright with lap at right angles to back, or leans slightly forward, or lies on her side.	Mother sits semi-reclined (not one degree of body slope but a range) – not on her side, never lying flat or almost flat on her back.
Mother often stuck in one position; often sacrifices her own comfort for "correct" latch; head, neck, and shoulders unsupported; her shoulders often unbalanced and/or hunched.	Mother has freedom of movement with the potential for complete body support, including head, neck, shoulders, upper back, lower back, and legs.
One maternal forearm and hand must hold the baby; the other hand often holds her breast.	Mother has at least one hand free; often both hands are free. Maternal arms often lie lightly on or loosely encircle the baby.
Mother must hold her baby, applying constant back pressure; this pressure often extends to the baby's neck or head.	Mother's body holds her baby. Sometimes she holds baby's bottom. Sometimes the baby's head rests on mother's arms.
Baby is held in one of three positions: cradle, cross-cradle, or rugby/football hold.	Mother's breast is round. There are potentially 360 baby positions.
There is a predetermined way to approach the breast; dorsal pressure keeps baby at breast level; baby approaches the breast from below.	Like the hands of a clock, the baby can approach the breast from any angle (above or below the breast), no dorsal pressure.

Constant dorsal pressure keeps baby close but there is often a gap or angle formed between the mother's and baby's bodies.	Baby lies tummy on mummy, with no gap or angle between baby's and mother's bodies; there is constant close ventral contact.
Baby lies vertically parallel (side-lying) or at right angles to the mother's body, i.e., transverse lie across her midriff.	Baby sometimes lies on top and across the mother's body (transverse lie) but usually in longitudinal or oblique lie.
Baby's legs and feet are loosely or poorly applied to mother's body; feet often only in contact with thin air.	Baby's thighs, calves, feet tops, and soles are touching and closely applied to the mother's body, or the furniture, or bed clothes, etc.
The first point of breast contact is the chin; baby's mouth gapes and lower lip is below the lower half of the areola (asymmetrical latch).	Baby often head bobs; the trigeminal area including the glabella are often the first point of breast contact (symmetrical latch).
Mothers are taught to wait for wide mouth gape and then latch or attach the baby onto the breast.	Babies often self-attach; when they don't, mothers help.

Reflex Activity or Hunger and Interest?

Hunger and interest are common watchwords characterising breastfeeding initiation. Faced with latch failure, or if the baby falls asleep at the breast, health professionals and mothers alike often say that the baby is not hungry or not interested in breastfeeding. In view of the strong reflex component stimulating breastfeeding observed during episodes of biological nurturing, we must address these interpretations.

The Role of Hunger in Frontal Feeding

First, hunger is not the only neonatal drive to breastfeed. Let us recall that healthy term infants are born well-fed and during the first 24 hours they only ingest small amounts of milk.[42] This does not mean that hunger never regulates feeding behaviours; rather, I suggest that babies latch on and breastfeed for a variety of reasons in different situations.

Babies who are allowed to remain lying prone but at a physiological body tilt on top of their mother's body go rapidly in and out of drowsy and sleep states. This is often called indeterminate sleep. In my study, compelling video data show how they often latch on or re-latch while asleep, even after 30 to 45 minutes of good milk transfer characterised by sucking bursts and audible swallowing. Independent of hunger, babies will often latch again and again in response to positional or endogenous stimuli that release feeding reflexes.

The BN approach helps condition the reflexes earlier. During the first days, the baby is learning how to coordinate sucking and swallowing with breathing for the first time. When the healthy term baby is at the right address, it usually does not take long to achieve reflex conditioning and physiological coordination, suggesting that this is best done before maternal milk volume increases (approximately the third postnatal day) and hunger increasingly becomes a factor.

Likewise, biological nurturing research rejects the common notion that reluctance or failure to latch indicates that the baby is not interested in breastfeeding. One way to trigger a latch is by releasing the foot reflexes, such as the Babinski and plantar grasp. This strong foot-to-mouth association was fascinating to observe. For example, when mothers wanted to put their sleeping babies down, they often checked to see if the baby was finished by spontaneously stroking the baby's feet. Of course, this was easy to do. They usually had both hands free because they did not need to hold the baby.

Neonatal interest can be defined as the amount of time during which the baby has focused attention on a stimulus.[43] "Interest," therefore, can only occur during a quiet alert behavioural state. For example, when the baby looks at bright lights, tracks bright objects like a red ball with his eyes, or gazes intently upon his mother's face. During the first three postnatal days, these times of focused attention are precious, promoting reciprocal behaviours like mimicry, mutual sensorial discovery, and communication. Babies are known to spend 75% to 80% of their time sleeping, moving rapidly from one state to the next so that, comparatively, these quiet alert times do not last very long during the first three postnatal days.

These facts suggest that "interest in breastfeeding" is not the right turn of phrase. Furthermore, when health professionals suggest that the baby is "not interested" in breastfeeding, it can undermine a mother's confidence, making her think that her baby does not like her milk or that she does not have enough. This can lead to feelings of guilt and inadequacy, which are heightened when the baby rapidly glugs the artificial milk drink in the bottle that is often given to the baby who is "disinterested" in breastfeeding. Taken together these facts and observations suggest, with a degree of certainty, that the mechanisms underpinning breastfeeding initiation are associated with simple reflex activity, not interest.

An example can help to clarify the misunderstanding about eliciting a reflex versus interest. The knee jerk reflex is a simple response mediated in the spinal cord and similar to many PNRs. The knee jerk is also used as a screening test to assess neurological function across the lifespan. When a doctor, using a patella hammer, attempts to elicit the knee jerk reflex and the knee does not respond, he does not suggest that it's because the knee is "not interested" in jerking. The doctor does not suggest waiting three hours to try again!

All nurses know that simple reflexes are assessed across behavioural states. For example, nurses are taught how to assess reflex activity in the unconscious patient. In the same way, when babies are in light sleep and drowsy states in BN positions, the inevitable body brushing releases the motor and searching PNRs. When the baby is sleeping, the reflex actions releasing self-attachment are somewhat blunted, reducing the strength and amplitude of the reflex response. Nevertheless, these mechanisms produce latch just as the doctor using the patella hammer produces the knee jerk.

In addition, we can certainly state that "interest" is not central to a successful transition from foetus to neonate. However, what is fundamental is early and frequent suckling and breast emptying during the first three days. Early and frequent suckling ensure a successful postnatal adaptation for healthy term babies. Early and frequent suckling keep the baby at the right address, protect the baby against infection, keep him warm, and ensure the tactile, olfactory, and eye-to-eye contact crucial to brain development. Early and frequent suckling help to maintain blood glucose concentrations at just the right levels. As described earlier, metabolically, when babies breastfeed frequently, they generate ketone bodies, an alternative source of fuel for the neonatal brain.[44] Research clearly demonstrates that the earlier babies latch on and suckle, the easier it is to establish breastfeeding.[45]

If early breastfeeding initiation has to do with releasing and conditioning reflexes – as the biological nurturing research data suggest – then we must consider eliminating the words "interest" and "hunger" from our vocabulary during the time of breastfeeding initiation.

CHAPTER 10

Mother's Breastfeeding Postures

One surprise in our study was that the position the mother sits in – mother's breastfeeding posture – was central to the release of the primitive neonatal reflexes (PNRs) as stimulants. Yet, that is what our observations suggested. Once we realised this, we needed to come up with a whole new set of research definitions.

Operational definitions are those used during a research investigation. These definitions are usually predetermined, enhancing the objectivity and reliability of the description. In the PhD study, however, the flexibility inherent in the descriptive design made it possible to identify and operationalise other ingredients or components identified at any time during the investigation. This enabled us to describe and define an unanticipated versatility in maternal breastfeeding positions.

We, therefore, spent hours studying the video clips using both slow/fast motion and pausing techniques to capture still pictures. Luckily two members of the PhD expert group had specialised knowledge from other disciplines. The National Childbirth Trust (NCT) lactation consultant was originally qualified as a structural engineer and the cranial osteopath was trained to make fine calculations comparing anatomical structures. In consultation with the supervisory panel, it was therefore possible to formulate, in retrospect, approximate, but concrete and measurable, angles of maternal body slope, quantifying a range of maternal postures.

Breastfeeding Postures: Research Definitions

At the time of my doctoral work, fixed rules concerning the mother's position, the baby's position, and breast attachment were considered to be the most important variables enabling pain-free effective breastfeeding.[1-3] Inch clarified the difference between breast positioning and breast attachment in the literature.[4] Although it is clear that these terms refer to the neonate, confusion can result from using the word "position" for both mother and baby. Therefore, for my study, we used the word *posture* to refer to the mother's position, whereas the word *position* always referred to the baby.

For the breastfeeding mothers who experienced latch refusal, sore nipples, or any other problems during the videotaped session, baby positions and postural changes were suggested after about five minutes and the videotape captured both before and after episodes. When we compared these episodes, we found striking differences in anatomical postural support. To clarify these differences, we need to look at the bony pelvis.

The Role of the Bony Pelvis

Kapandji, a French orthopaedic surgeon, integrated and illustrated complex physiology and mechanical functioning of joints and muscles within the anatomical context. His explanations and illustrations, together with those from recent British midwifery textbooks, provide the basis for understanding the difference between upright and laid-back sitting postures.[5]

The Bony Pelvis

The bony pelvis is literally a pivotal system supporting the abdomen. It houses the reproductive organs and links the vertebral column to the legs. Transmitting gravitational forces from the vertebral column to the lower limbs, the pelvis comprises four bony parts and three joints: two sacroiliac and the symphysis pubis joint. The coccyx, the lowest part of the spine, articulates with the sacrum, a triangular-shaped bone composed of five fused sacral vertebrae vertically wedged between two iliac bones, sometimes called innominate bones, which are paired and symmetrical.

The iliac bones comprise three parts: the ilia or wing-like upper crests that extend to and fuse with the pubis, thus forming two-fifths of the upper border of the acetabulum, the point of femoral articulation. The ischia, each extending from the acetabulum above, form a downward projection or protuberance of rounded bony mass below, called ischial tuberosities. The pubis is a small bone, linking the ilia anteriorly and forming one-fifth of the anterior acetabulum.

The sacrum, suspended from the iliac bones by ligaments, forms "a self-locking system," whereby the greater the weight, the more tightly it locks. See Figure 15, which illustrates these parts of the bony pelvis. Sacral movement is achieved through the sacroiliac joints with a relatively limited range. Sacral nutation, coming from the Latin *nutare*, meaning to nod, refers to a complex system of sacral forward and backward rotational movements.[6] See Figure 16, which illustrates sacral rotation.

Figure 15: The Bony Pelvis

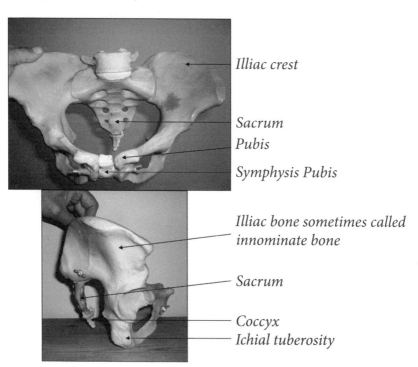

Illiac crest

Sacrum
Pubis
Symphysis Pubis

Illiac bone sometimes called innominate bone

Sacrum

Coccyx
Ichial tuberosity

Figure 16: Sacral Nutation

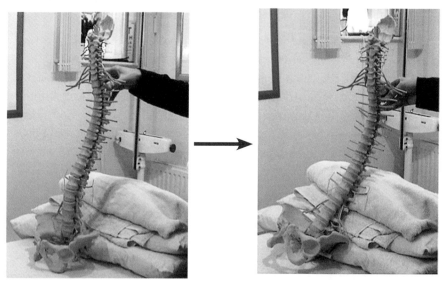

Upright Ischial Sitting   *Laid-back Sacral Sitting*

Pelvic Sitting Support

When sitting bolt upright, or leaning slightly forward, the body mass is supported evenly by the two ischial tuberosities. In ischial sitting postures – for example, those used to drive a car, ride a bike, or to work at the computer – the weight of the trunk sits firmly upon a solid base, either a chair, or a seat. Strictly speaking, it is irrelevant if the base has a back since a chair back only limits the potential to recline. However, having a back support may add feelings of security. Body weight is placed equally on both ischial tuberosities. The seat is at a height that permits the thighs to be parallel to the floor and the feet rest flat on the floor. The body leans forward from the hips when necessary but does not curve at the shoulders or neck.[7]

This is the sitting posture that is normally termed "correct" for breast-feeding. The body is aligned from the hips up, just as when standing "correctly." Interestingly, Kapandji calls this "correct" postural position the "typist's position," characterising it as fraught with potential for muscular fatigue. The typist's posture is the most difficult body posture to sustain.[8]

In contrast, when sitting laid-back, for example, sprawled on a chair or sofa while watching television, the back of the chair or sofa always supports the shoulders and torso. Bony pelvic reliance comprises the posterior surface of the sacrum and the coccyx with limited ischial support. Kapandji terms this posture the "position of relaxation." It is neither sitting nor lying down but "achieved with the help of cushions or specially designed chairs." Figure 17 compares and contrasts bony pelvic reliance, depicting an adaptation of Kapandji's "typist's position" and his "position of relaxation".[9]

Having understood these bony postural facts, and the small but important range of potential maternal pelvic movement, it became straightforward to define maternal posture using three parameters: degree of recline or body slope, bony pelvic reliance, and body support. Definitions determining the scientific angle of recline are summarised in Figure 18 and the operational definitions used during the PhD study are shown in the table below.

Table 4: Operational Definitions for Maternal Posture

	Degree of recline	Bony pelvic reliance	Body support
Upright sitting	>74°	Ischial	Head, neck, shoulders, upper back do not touch seatback
Laid-back sitting	15° to 74°	Coccyx or sacral	Head, neck, upper back firmly against seatback
Flat/side-lying	0° to 14°	None	Head, neck, torso against bed or thin pillow

Figure 19 illustrates these definitions in the flesh. Observe how the bottle-feeding mother below on the left is ischial sitting, upright at 90°, as is the breastfeeding mother in the middle. On the right, the same breastfeeding mother has changed to sacral sitting and is semi-reclined at a 35° angle.

Postures and Breastfeeding Duration: Research Results

The 40 mothers in my doctoral study tried biological nurturing with varying maternal body slope (all of them tried it at least on one occasion when being videotaped). At six postnatal weeks, all were breastfeeding – 87.5% (*n*=35) exclusively. The 100% rate of breastfeeding duration occurred

Figure 17: Bony Pelvic Reliance

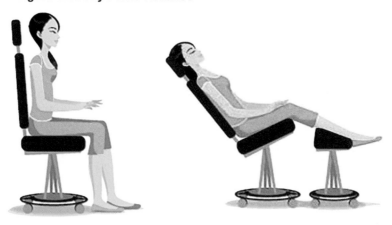

From the 1980s to today, British text books have suggested that midwives show mothers the "correct" upright breastfeeding posture, the most difficult body posture to sustain.

Figure 18: Calculating the angle of recline

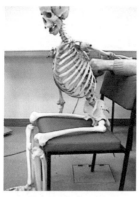

The long axis of the mother's body was defined by an imaginary line traced from the maternal sternal notch to her pubic bone (line A to B). The sternal notch was chosen because it was more visible than the mother's spine. The angle formed at the junction between the long part of the mother's body and the horizontal axis was measured using a protractor. To simplify the calculation, 0° on the protractor was selected rather than 180° to mark the flat or side-lying angle (parallel to the horizontal axis). These definitions, formulated in retrospect, were approximate due to the inevitable camera distortion found in the pictures.

Mother leaning forward ≈115°

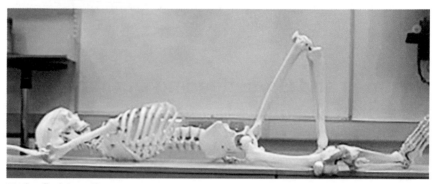

Mother flat lying ≈0°

despite more than a quarter of the mothers (*n*=11) having had a caesarean birth. This result needs to be interpreted with caution, as some would suggest that it implies cause and effect, whereas there is no such intent.

Another factor that could account for increased breastfeeding rates is that a breastfeeding assessment was carried out by whoever was available. Mothers self-reported. Partners and parents commented. Although I was only present as an observer and a research midwife, access to the various hospitals had been negotiated with the view that mothers and babies would remain safe under my care. I made professional evaluations of latch and milk transfer, although these were only shared verbally with the mother if and when needed.

Nevertheless, I hold strong beliefs in every mother's capacity to breast-feed. Perhaps my convictions were transmitted in tacit ways and we must ask the question: are the beliefs and attitudes of the health professional integral to their breastfeeding assessment and/or a mother's success?

Figure 19: Dorsal Breastfeeding Positions

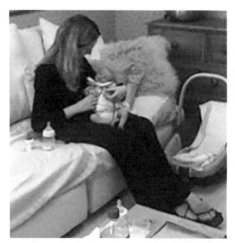
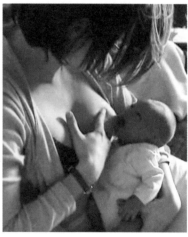

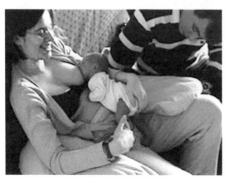

In the flesh, therefore, the bottle-feeding mother above on the left is ischial sitting, upright at 90° as is the breastfeeding mother on the right.

On the left, the same breastfeeding mother has changed to sacral sitting and is semi-reclined at a 35° angle.

My personal convictions may have influenced the mothers. Some would suggest that this personal component is integral to breastfeeding support and is just as important as any other ingredient of an intervention.

A key finding was that more PNRs were observed as breastfeeding stimulants, aiding latch and sustaining milk transfer when mothers sat laid-back than when they sat upright or lay on their sides, and this difference was statistically significant.[10] One mother, without any problems, wanted to be filmed trying out breastfeeding like in the *Delivery Self-Attachment* video.[11] Towards the end of the study, five mothers shared their problems or concerns with me before I filmed the first episode. For those five mothers, I suggested that they try BN mother postures. Problems such as sore nipples (*n*=3), backache (*n*=1), and latch refusal (*n*=1) were immediately improved.

Does This Mean That Mothers Should Never Initiate Breastfeeding in Upright Postures?

Human mothers and babies are extremely versatile, able to breastfeed in many different positions, and it would not be helpful to prescribe laid-back postures as the only way to initiate breastfeeding. Observations for the first episode demonstrated that 12 of the 27 breastfeeding mothers who sat upright latched their baby successfully onto the breast with good milk transfer. However, only a quarter of them (*n*=3) were pain-free. The other nine mothers modified their baby's positions, their own postures, or both, in subsequent episodes to achieve an increase in comfort.

Likewise, three of the four mothers who started the feed lying on their sides latched the baby successfully with good milk transfer. However, side-lying was not sustainable for two of the four mothers who subsequently changed posture: one said she had sore nipples, and another said she had backache. That meant that 11 mothers (over 25% of the sample) breastfed through pain during the first episode. These findings replicate Sulcova's observations of postural discomfort (see box).

Grey Literature

In PhD research, Sulcova (1997), a behavioural psychologist, reports maternal feeding observations in descriptions of spontaneous mother/baby behaviours. This "mother/baby choreography" underpinned the Prague Newborn Behaviour Description Technique, an assessment instrument that provides information on the healthy newborn's level of well-being through observations of maternal/infant behavioural interactions. As a component, Sulcova observed the breastfeeding techniques of mothers who were taught positioning and attachment skills, either sitting upright or side-lying. Sulcova describes tension-laden and unbalanced maternal sitting postures, suggesting that mothers will always sacrifice their personal and positional comfort for a good latch.[12]

The mother who wanted to try out the "breast crawl" using the positions she saw in the *Delivery Self-Attachment* video was an experienced mother having her second baby. Following a home birth, she had no breastfeeding difficulties. Interestingly, she had seen the video[13] some years prior to this pregnancy but had never tried it. She expressed a desire to lie flat to see if the baby would self-attach (like the ones in the video). Interestingly, after about three minutes, her baby had not attached, and she asked me what to do. I suggested that she participate, and she shifted her baby's position, placing him on the breast, at which time he self-attached immediately, but she is recorded on the research videotape saying that she prefers upright sitting.

However, following completion of the postnatal questionnaire (at six weeks), she subsequently sent me a personal VHS videotape, recorded by her husband, demonstrating how her baby, in full BN baby positions but flat-lying mother postures, self-attached, indicating that she had tried this again. I feel that her initial experience needs to be registered as she was the only mother who, having tried more reclined postures, is recorded to prefer being upright.

Below are some questions and comments I've received on the issue of traditional breastfeeding positions versus BN.

Question

I am a Student Breastfeeding Counsellor and have been following and researching your work on BN for a few months now… I just wondered what you think BN means for more traditional positions, and is there a place for both or do you think BN is the ultimate way forward? As a student BFC who will be helping women in the future, I just want to figure out what BN means for me and the way I "teach" in the future.

My Response

I think that mothers and babies are extremely versatile, able to breastfeed in a variety of positions, and this is perhaps what makes us different from other mammals. Nevertheless, I wonder if BN maternal positions are more species-specific in that the amount of body space available to accommodate the movements of the neonate is increased when mother leans back. In traditional positions, the baby usually lies across the midriff because the body is closed, whereas in BN, babies lie longitudinally or obliquely. We have a relatively small midriff compared to, say, a polar bear, whose babies often feed vertically, but polar bears also use a variety of positions.

Question

I am a student breastfeeding counsellor (BFC) with the NCT. A question that I didn't have the opportunity to ask after your presentation: do you find that babies who are started on breastfeeding along biological nurturing lines, go on to feed in more "conventional" positions, lying across the mother's lap, for example? I sort of presumed that once they'd been allowed to find the nipple and initiate breastfeeding on their own natural terms, they would later be more flexible about different positions, but I'd be really interested to know if this is so. I would love to teach couples about this approach to breastfeeding, but I can already hear women telling me that they want to be able to feed their babies while out and about, and it's very hard to recline comfortably on a park bench or cafe chair!

My Response

It does not take long for the reflexes to become conditioned and then mothers use a variety of positions. Sometimes they lean back just a bit when they are out as many find this comfortable. BN maternal postures can be more upright and still use gravity positively. It is just when mothers are bolt upright that gravity often works against latch. Nevertheless, once the reflexes are conditioned, it usually does not make any difference at all. When mothers are out and about, they can use any position that is comfortable.

Comment

I'm very encouraged by what you've said – it makes sense that babies adapt to different positions once they've established breastfeeding, I suppose. It doesn't make evolutional sense to be too inflexible, after all. I was really so struck by BN, and can't wait to try it out myself, but knew that mothers would want to know how it worked for them after the first early weeks.

In summary, posture is a dynamic variable, changing often to enhance enjoyment and meet our needs no matter what we are doing. There is a strong argument suggesting that people will continue to do the things they enjoy, and this makes maternal comfort during breastfeeding a key issue in breastfeeding duration.

Maternal Comfort Mechanisms

All mothers experience a wide range of challenges to their personal comfort right after birth. The abrupt change in body shape can be a real shock and sometimes body parts feel sensitive, ache, or are sore. This can be compounded by abdominal pain if the mother has had a caesarean birth, or perineal pain if she has had an episiotomy or an operative or assisted delivery. Breastfeeding often exacerbates discomfort as breasts and nipples can hurt, and many mothers complain of neck tension and shoulder pain as it is difficult to maintain the "typist's position" for long periods of time.

Laid-back breastfeeding, by definition, means that every part of the mother's body – importantly, her head, neck, shoulders, upper, and lower back – are supported and relaxed. Mothers often say that as soon as they sit back, the shoulder and neck tension melt away. Nipple pain is often alleviated immediately, and this may happen because gravity is not dragging the baby down the upright maternal midriff. Mothers also have increased freedom of movement as one or both hands are free. Their bodies hold the baby not their arms. Figure 20 compares maternal body support in upright postures with BN.

Read what one student midwife wrote:

> I am fascinated by the BN approach, but I have never before put into practice your ideas. Until now! I attended a new mum on a postnatal visit at home who was experiencing problems with latching and sore nipples. When I arrived, she seemed a bit distressed and her baby was crying, so I suggested we try something different to what she had been shown by the midwives. I asked her to semi-recline and popped baby on her chest and within about 3 minutes she self-attached and the mother was totally amazed and had no pain at all on feeding.

My mentor who was with me commented on how she had never seen anything like it. Thank you for your insight.

Angie, Student Midwife (now qualified) and
breastfeeding counsellor, Bournemouth, England

Psychological Comfort: Protecting the Frontal Region of the Body

Breastfeeding is both a private and a social act. Initially, privacy often gives mothers the space to experiment in a state of undress, but very soon they become eager to share their excitement and experiences with anyone who will listen. One of the reasons why mother-to-mother support and peer groups work so well is that most mothers just love talking about their babies. While they're talking, they are also breastfeeding and seeing other mothers who are breastfeeding. This can lead to intimate sharing or debriefing, offering psychological comfort.

One topic that is consistently discussed in these groups is how to breast-feed discreetly. Many mothers express a physical as well as a psychological discomfort about bearing breasts and torso in public.

Figure 20: Maternal Body Support from Upright to BN postures

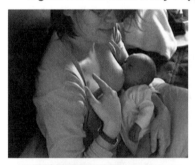
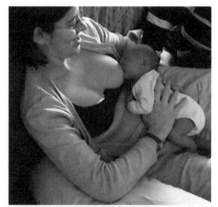
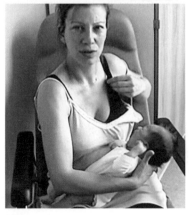
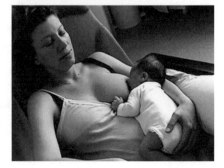

The frontal region (the area from the sternum to the pubis) of the human body is an extremely sensitive area and may play an important role in close physical relationships. That may explain why so many mothers feel exposed even thinking about their frontal region being undressed or unprotected. But the need to protect this area is relatively common for anyone in an unfamiliar social situation.

Desmond Morris observes that when people feel threatened or unsafe, they often send unconscious but defensive body barrier signals that cover the frontal region of the body.[14] Morris illustrates that when diplomats arrive in a foreign country, they take measures to conceal or protect this body area. Prior to greeting a public figure on foreign territory, a woman dignitary may reach across her body to her purse, making a temporary bar across the front torso, whereas a man may straighten his cuff links, bringing both hands in front of his body. Both may extend one arm across the body while shaking hands.

This need to protect the frontal body region in public situations may be an unconscious reason motivating many mothers to sit upright to breastfeed, diminishing the space that is visible and holding the baby across their midriff when they are out, at home with visitors, or when people take photos. In any case, once the reflexes are conditioned, the degree of body slope is less important. Furthermore, there is not one ideal degree of body slope, and when mothers are in more "public" situations it is still possible to use gravity positively by leaning back into a comfortable sitting posture reliant upon both ischial and sacral support.

Figure 21: Biological Nurturing When Out and About

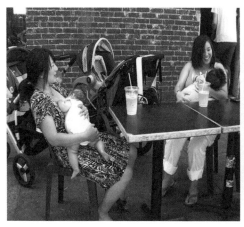
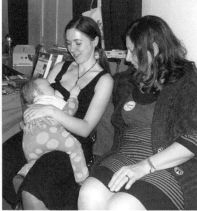

The baby's position lies differently in biological nurturing positions. In Figure 21, in the photo on the left, you see Elaine Scully, sitting next to me after a public conference. She has no difficulty protecting her torso. Read below how she now shares BN positions with other mothers. Likewise, the mothers in the café are also practising BN discreetly. Notice how all their babies lie obliquely across their bodies, similar to the way Morris describes women dignitaries reaching across their bodies. Biological nurturing baby positions add a natural cover, protecting a mother's physical as well as psychological comfort.

◆

ELAINE'S TESTIMONIAL

A few days after the conference, I met a new mum at our café who was already sitting in the biological nurturing position with her son asleep on her. As she told me their history and how much of a struggle feeding was, I used a doll to show her how from where she is, she could latch her baby on, and then when he woke up, she tried it.

Mum exclaimed with joy! She wanted to know why no one else had ever told her about this as, when her baby had struggled at the start, the hospital had told her to use a very mechanical "holding breast and baby's head and forcing together" method. He fed like a dream after using BN.

From there, I've gone on to promoting BN to many mothers with babies and antenatally. I knew of BN before but after the conference I felt far better equipped to suggest it to others.

◆

In the next chapter, we explore in depth how the baby's lie, or the direction of his or her position varies, personalising each baby's latch.

CHAPTER 11

Baby's Breastfeeding Postures

An overall aim of biological nurturing is to facilitate the processes of adaptation by highlighting the points of continuity from womb to world, as discussed previously. These connections between foetus and neonate are inherent in the components and mechanisms of biological nurturing and have immediate implications for clinical support. For example, we saw that primitive neonatal reflexes (PNRs) develop from 28 gestational weeks. At birth, the baby relies upon these familiar movements to find the breast, latch on and feed. In this chapter, we discuss how retaining two components of foetal position helps to facilitate the transition from womb feeding to breastfeeding.

When lying prone in a physiological body tilt on top of the gentle maternal body slope, the baby often moves into a position similar to how he was lying in the womb (albeit usually head up). This point of continuity leads to further clarification of the lie and the attitude, the two characteristics of the newborn's position that remain similar from foetus to neonate.

What is Lie?

Simply put, lie is the direction of the baby's position. I have borrowed the term from the obstetrical or midwifery assessments of "foetal lie" made during antenatal visits. Foetal lie is formally defined as a relation between the long axis of the baby's body to the long axis of the mother's womb.[1] Foetal lie may be longitudinal, oblique, or transverse (see Figure 22).

During the last trimester of gestation, the foetus normally lies head down in a longitudinal or oblique direction. A transverse foetal lie at term is a

Figure 22: Foetal Lie

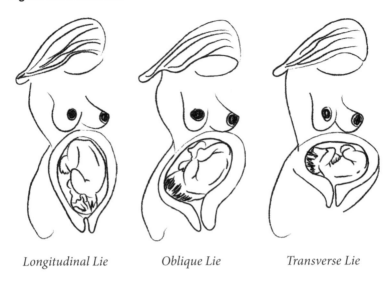

Longitudinal Lie *Oblique Lie* *Transverse Lie*

malposition, and the incidence is one in 300 to 400.[2,3] If a transverse lie is sustained during labour, it leads to a malpresentation. The baby's shoulder is usually the presenting part. The mother will require a caesarean section.

When I understood how important it is to assess lie in the breastfeeding context, I formally defined the term and started teaching it to my students. Building upon definitions of foetal lie, neonatal lie is the relation between the long axis (spinal column) of the baby to the long axis (spinal column) of the mother. In biological nurturing positions, you can identify three positional directions: longitudinal, transverse, and oblique (see Figure 23).

My breastfeeding data suggest that many babies root, head bob, and self-attach spontaneously as soon as they move into the familiar positional direction. In other words, continuity of lie from foetus to neonate appears to support spontaneous latch. However, breastfeeding in upright positions usually forces the baby into a transverse lie.

The mechanisms are easy to understand. When a mother sits upright to breastfeed, she maintains her back at right angles to her lap. This approximate 90° angle closes her body, limiting the space available to her baby. This may explain why midwives have always taught mothers to hold their babies in one of three positions: cradle, cross-cradle, or rugby position. No matter which hold she uses, the lie is transverse. When the mother is told to bring her baby in close, she has little choice. The baby usually only fits at right angles to her body. This means that the baby inevitably lies in a transverse position across or by his mother's midriff (see Figure 24).

Figure 23: Neonatal Lie

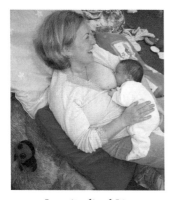

Longitudinal Lie

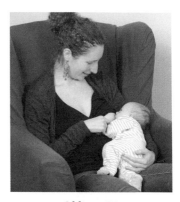

Oblique Lie

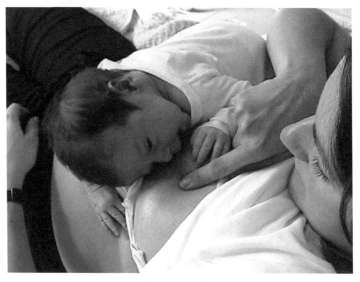

Transverse Lie

In other words, when the mother sits upright to breastfeed her one-day-old baby, he lies in a position that was considered "abnormal" yesterday. This abrupt change in positional direction from foetus to neonate may be at the root of some of the early latch problems mothers often experience. We must recall that over a third of mothers who stop breastfeeding during the first postnatal week say they couldn't get their baby to latch.[4]

In contrast, as soon as a mother leans back, the dimensions of her body space increase – particularly her midriff, or the space between the sternal notch and her pubic bone. The round breast now is available on an open

Figure 24: Transverse lie in upright postures

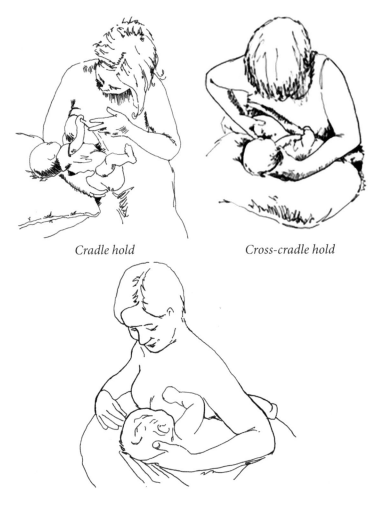

Cradle hold   *Cross-cradle hold*

Rugby hold

plane. The baby often modifies the lie, or direction of his position, using the motor reflexes released by positional brushing with the mother's body. More babies will spontaneously adopt a longitudinal or oblique lie because these are the normal foetal positions.

Indeed, a real advantage to BN is that babies can manoeuvre around the breast, like the hands of a clock, therefore approaching the areola from any direction. Anytime there are latching problems or sore nipples, modifications to the baby's lie can be made quickly and easily by suggesting that the mother rests her back and head against the back of the chair or sofa. As she leans back, she instantly opens her body. She may intuitively place her baby or baby may manoeuvre himself into a familiar positional direction. Babies often latch spontaneously.

Close examination of the biological nurturing data suggests those newborn babies who were in a longitudinal or oblique foetal lie may find a transverse lie awkward, difficult, or even painful, and this has to do with the baby's degree of flexion or what midwives call "the attitude."

What is Neonatal Attitude?

Neonatal attitude is the second subcomponent of the baby's biological nurturing position. Again, I have borrowed the term from obstetrical and/ or midwifery antenatal assessments. Foetal attitude is formally defined as the relation between the baby's limbs and head to his body.[5] In simple terms, attitude is the degree of flexion and ranges from fully flexed to completely extended (see Figure 25). When the foetus is fully flexed, his head and spine are curved inward with arms crossed over his chest, thighs, and calves drawn upward, ankles often crossed. This is the optimal position for labour. The baby forms a compact egg shaped oval. Birth will likely be spontaneous.

Even though a longitudinal lie is optimal, babies can still have their heads, backs, and/or legs fully or partially extended (for example, a baby in a posterior position where the baby's back faces the mother's back, or in a breech, face, or brow presentation). In any case, the foetal attitude has an

Figure 25: Foetal Attitude

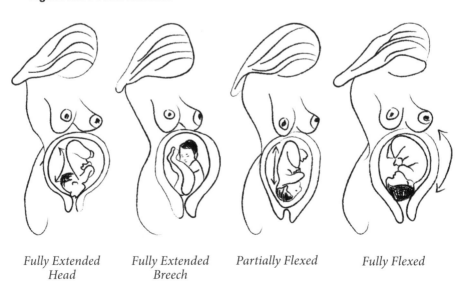

Fully Extended   Fully Extended   Partially Flexed   Fully Flexed
Head   Breech

impact upon the degree of flexion or extension during latch.

Anyone can assess a newborn baby's lie and attitude, yet few health professionals are taught to do this. That's because biological nurturing is a new approach that challenges traditional beliefs about the "correct" latch. The BN latch is described differently from the "asymmetrical" and "correct" latch depicted in the mainstream breastfeeding literature. In BN, there's great diversity of lie and attitude. As described above, prior to the introduction of BN, the transverse lie usually characterised the "normal" breastfeeding position. Traditionally, mothers were instructed to gently flex their babies around their midriffs, regardless of baby's foetal attitude. In the three traditional breastfeeding holds, the baby usually approached the breast from below. BN changes things and Figure 26 illustrates the versatility of BN lie and attitude.

Look closely at Figure 26. You will see the different positional directions or ways to approach the breast as well as some reflexes. The baby on the right is about to turn her head to the midline. She is in a transverse lie in partial flexion. She looks like a swimmer taking a breath, doing the freestyle crawl. Her head is turned to her left, the head-turning reflex will bring it into the midline, so she can latch.

The baby, in a longitudinal lie in partial extension, is just about to brush

Figure 26: Versatility of Fetal Lie and Attitude.

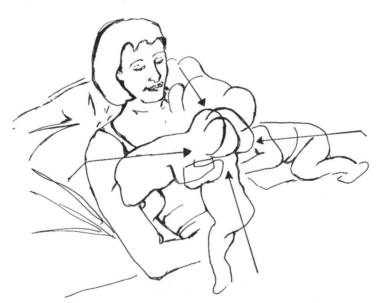

the top of his foot against the bed releasing the placing reflex, which will push him up mum's body. And the baby lying over the mother's shoulder has been born by caesarean section. Lying obliquely in partial extension, his mother doesn't have to worry about her baby kicking or moving against her fresh wound. The last baby, approaching the breast from the left, is head bobbing in a transverse lie and partially extended. The soles of his feet are against the bed, aiding positional stability.

Biological nurturing turns latch assessment upside down! The versatility of the BN positions requires new assessment techniques. I introduce the concept of "good fit" to meet this need.

What is Good Fit?

All mammals have biological strategies that enable mothers' and babies' bodies to fit together to accomplish those physiological acts that ensure the survival of the species (for example, grooming, protection, transportation, and feeding). I call this good fit and Figure 27 illustrates some of these strategies.

Figure 27: The Concept of Good Fit

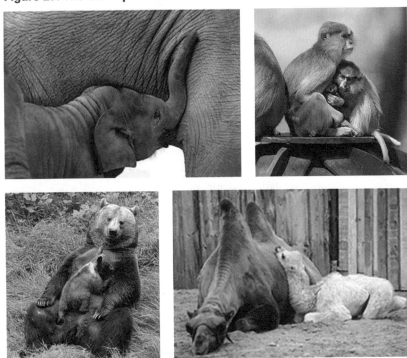

Good fit is species-specific and goes hand in hand with the mammalian habitat. As we discussed in Chapter 5, when mothers keep their babies at the right address, the mother's body and lactational apparatus provide what Alberts calls that natal environment conducive to "learning as a property of a behaving body".[6] Learning is reciprocal because mothers' and babies' bodies fit together like the pieces of a jigsaw.

Biological nurturing finely tunes this compact body-to-body fit through continuous ventral, full-frontal contact. When the human baby lies prone but tilted upwards on a gentle maternal body slope, good fit describes how well the baby's face and BN position are synchronised with his mother's breast and body.

I reiterate that the right breastfeeding address is on the breast, with baby either suckling or sleeping cheek to breast. We have already discussed one of the reasons that babies need to be located full on the mother's breast; our babies do not move easily or rapidly. Another reason is because our babies, unlike most other mammals, are born with cute, chubby, fat pads in their cheeks. Reciprocally, human mothers, unlike most other mammals, are endowed with varying amounts of adipose breast tissue.

Biological nurturing brings these two fatty tissues together. However, like their mothers' breasts, babies' faces come in all shapes and sizes. Some babies have square chins. Others are pointed or receding. The mission of a health professional supporting breastfeeding is to ensure that the fat pads of the baby's cheeks are closely applied to the adipose tissue of the mother's breast. This can release up to five of the baby's facial reflexes with eight releasing points.

The baby's face has two reflex diamonds: the Cardinal reflexes make a small lip diamond; and starting between the baby's eyes, the Glabella, Masseter (chin jerk), and exaggerated right and left rooting reflexes create a larger diamond. Together with the woodpecker reflex (head bobbing), these five reflexes comprise the trigeminal area of the baby's face, which is divided into three parts: ophthalmic, maxillary and mandibular. Figure 28 illustrates the eight reflex points included within these divisions.

Following a normal spontaneous birth, when the baby is at the right address in BN positions, his attitude is usually partially or fully flexed; the entire trigeminal area of the baby's face is stimulated with each head bob; the latch is usually symmetrical.

In contrast, a hyperextended attitude often characterises a malposition during gestation, or suggests a preterm or small for gestational age baby. While latching, a hyperextended neonate often leads in with his chin,

Figure 28: The Reflex Diamonds

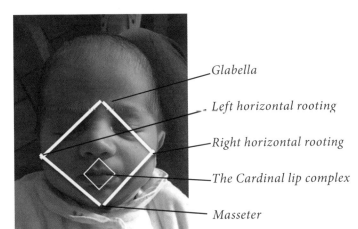

Glabella

Left horizontal rooting

Right horizontal rooting

The Cardinal lip complex

Masseter

spontaneously triggering the Masseter chin jerk reflex releasing mandibular movement; his latch will likely be asymmetrical.

Importantly, the Masseter reflex is always implicated in milk transfer. The Masseter is a primary feeding reflex. The chin taps the breast to release jaw movement promoting those rhythmic suckling bursts associated with successful milk transfer that Mike Woolridge identified so many years ago.[7]

Now let's apply some of these observations to clinical practice. Look at Figure 29.

The attitude of the newborn on the left is one of full flexion suggesting that the ophthalmic, maxillary, and mandibular trigeminal facial divisions will be stimulated simultaneously; his latch is likely to be symmetrical. Some lactation consultants might say that he's nipple sucking. But this latch, when

Figure 29: Assessing Attitude at a Glance.

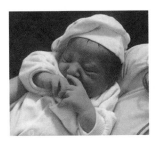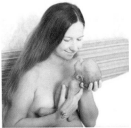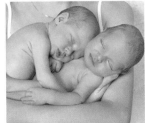

spontaneous, is usually pain-free and effective.

The baby in the middle is hyper-extended suggesting that she will stimulate the mandibular trigeminal facial division first, leading to an asymmetrical latch.

Finally, the twins in the last photo are a lovely illustration of good fit. They may be identical but their latch during the early days will likely be very different. The twin on the left is fully flexed and will probably latch like the baby in the first photo. Her sister, on the other hand, is partially extended so her head bobbing will likely stimulate the maxillary and mandibular trigeminal facial divisions. Even though her latch may exclude ophthalmic (glabella) stimulation, it will likely be a normal symmetrical latch.

In summary, lie and attitude are useful indicators of the baby's positional needs to achieve optimal attachment and can also help to verify gestational age.[8] In particular, observations of the baby's attitude appear to be strongly associated with the degree of latch symmetry, challenging current beliefs. Just as there are not three "correct" baby holds or two "correct" maternal postures, biological nurturing highlights that there's not one "correct asymmetrical" latch. The only correct latch is the one that works; the correct latch is pain free and provides good milk transfer. Anytime a mother is experiencing latching difficulties, your assessment of lie and attitude will help her shift her baby's position to ensure better fit.

CHAPTER 12

Lessons from Other Mammals

An understanding of the concept of good fit leads us to explore further the positions other mammals use to nurture their offspring.

Compare the pictures of a polar bear and a human mother in Figure 30; both are breastfeeding upright. Their babies are vertical. We do not need a tape measure to say that the distance in inches between the sternum and the pubis of the polar bear is greater than that of the human mother. Although they are quadrupeds, the cubs stand upright on two feet. The ground provides their feet with a broad, firm base, promoting positional stability. The cub on the left is hyperextended whereas his brother is partially

Figure 30: Mammals Breastfeeding Upright

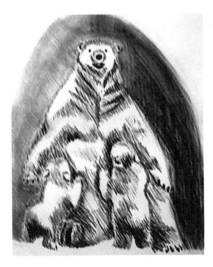
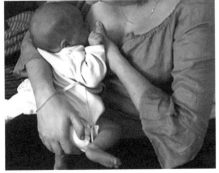

extended. The polar bear mother can feed in an upright posture without holding her babies, and therefore without applying pressure to their backs, necks, or heads. Vertical breastfeeding postures appear to work a treat for the polar bear. However, the upright human mother does have to hold her baby.

Although it is possible for the human neonate to breastfeed when held vertically in front of and parallel to the mother's torso, the small space does not accommodate the baby's flexed attitude. If the baby's attitude had been extended, mum could have placed her baby vertically straddling her thigh. This position is sometimes called the vertical football or koala hold and can work really well for babies whose foetal attitude was one of full extension.

For this baby, however, the position looks awkward and uncomfortable for both mother and baby. When the mother holds her baby upright, her arm pressure boxes the baby into her body, limiting neonatal movement and locomotion. The baby is somewhat stuck in the maternal midriff with feet unsupported. The mother struggles to provide positional stability.

It makes physiological sense that all mammals would have a biological strategy to provide their own positional stability. Human babies make use of inborn reflexes to anchor themselves to remain in place. But here, the baby is unable to move up or down. Therefore, the reflexes are suppressed, wasted, or expressed as barriers.

See how the neonate's feet and legs are in contact with thin air. Placing, stepping, and the sustained Babinski toe fan will not help this baby self attach or stabilise his position. Unlike the polar bear, when her baby is vertical, the human mother bears his full weight on her forearm. She must control latch and milk transfer, and she must also try to provide positional stability.

Now look at what happens in Figure 31, below, as soon as the mother sits more comfortably. Even a slight shift in posture seems to change everything. Mum's back now touches the sofa. Because she is fully supported, she can release the pressure against baby's back, although she keeps her hands lightly posed on her baby, similar to the ape mother in Figure 34 at the end of the chapter. Continuous close ventral contact is now possible. Baby lies on top of mum's body, first supporting just his legs and then supporting his feet against mum's thigh. The baby provides his own positional stability.

The above observations suggest that the optimal feeding position for the human baby is abdominal not dorsal, although, as said previously, mothers and babies are versatile, able to breastfeed in many different positions. Anatomical evidence supports this interpretation. At birth, the neonate's vertebral column is similar to those quadruped mammals whose offspring feed abdominally, that is, the human neonate has one single skeletal back

Figure 31: Biological Nurturing Laid-Back Postures

- *Open the mother's body*
- *Increase the dimensions of her torso*
- *Provide a gentle slope aiding neonatal locomotion*
- *Promote an up and down or oblique baby lie*
- *Promote maternal comfort, relaxation*
- *Optimise mother–baby eye-to-eye contact*

Mothers do not need to hold the baby applying back or neck pressure but they often make a body nest with their arms and spontaneously hold their baby's bottom.

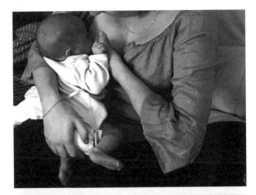
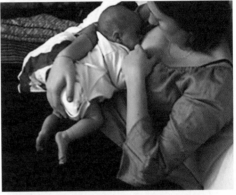
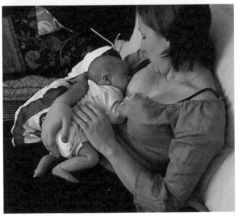

curvature or kyphosis. Jack Stern, an American expert in anatomy explains this below and with his permission, I adapted one of his figures to illustrate human spine development. See Figure 32.

In other words, contrary to their bipedal mothers, whose vertebral column is normally composed of two lordosi, human babies are quadrupeds at birth. They are born with a backbone similar to that of other quadrupeds,

Figure 32: Morphological Differences Between Human Mothers and Their Babies[1]

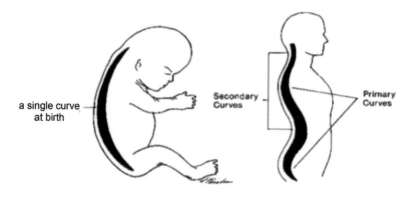

The baby's entire vertebral column has a gentle curve that is concave on its ventral surface... However, the newborn cervical and lumbar regions are soon lost. As the child begins to lift its head, and becoming accentuated when the child starts to sit erect, the intervertebral discs of the cervical region become thicker on their anterior margins and cause the cervical portion of the vertebral column to develop a gentle curve that is concave on its posterior surface. A posterior concavity is called a lordosis; thus, a cervical lordosis is a normal product of development. It can be eliminated by flexion of the neck. As the child begins to sit erect, and becoming accentuated as it starts to walk, the lumbar vertebrae and intervertebral discs become thickened at their anterior margins, inducing a lumbar lordosis. As in the neck, flexion of the lumbar column temporarily eliminates the lordosis.

such as rodents, dogs, and cats.

Alberts has carried out extensive studies examining the habitat and niche of the Norway rat. The dam feeds her pups in what Alberts calls an "arched-back nursing" posture and the litter (termed "the huddle") has close, continuous ventral contact with the ground or with another pup in the huddle.[2]

There is great diversity among mammals. They dwell on the land, in the sea, and in the air, and come in all shapes and sizes. We find mammalian mothers using arched-back nursing postures across a number of the land-dwelling orders. Many small mammals use an arched back nursing posture to feed their offspring, although pigs, who are hoofed mammals, also use it. However, this appears to be age-specific. Figure 33 displays some quadruped mammals in arched-back nursing postures.

Of course, we are primates, and like our closest cousins, apes and

Figure 33: Arched Back Nursing

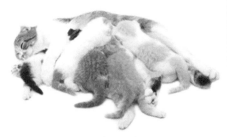
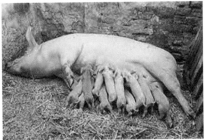

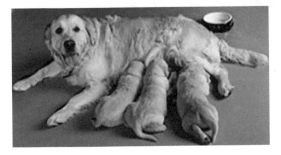
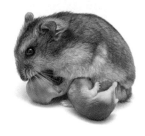

monkeys, we breastfeed in more vertical postures. Look at Figure 34. Although apes can walk on two feet, they are largely knuckle walkers. Both mother and baby are born, and remain, lifelong quadrupeds. And you can see the mother's single back curve, first in an upright maternal posture and then when she sits semi-reclined. When she is upright, her baby is vertical in a longitudinal lie. Apes have extremely strong grasping reflexes, and it is likely that grasping is the strategy that keeps baby close, maintaining his positional stability, because mum is not applying strong pressure on the baby's back. Taken together, these observations suggest that the baby's habitat, niche, and optimal feeding position within that habitat are strongly associated with his mother's morphology and also depends upon his maturity of locomotion.

In contrast, human mothers don't have that "gentle back curve that is concave on its ventral surface".[3] Human mothers are bipedal! These observations highlight a positional paradox that is uniquely human. Unlike other mammals, the vertebral structure of the human mother is different from her baby. Being upright is our human condition, and we are constantly struggling against gravity to accomplish our activities of daily living. For example, we eat sitting upright with our digestive tracts in perfect alignment. But the drive towards verticality has permeated many aspects of our

Figure 34: Order Primata

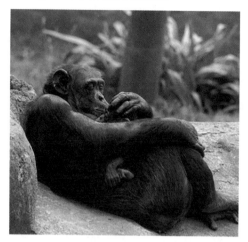 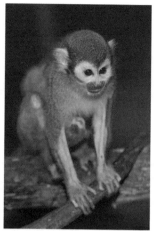

industrialised cultures. Culturally, in many societies, humans are regulated by a tacit upright morality.

If you look up the word "upright" in the dictionary, you will find a list of words highlighting moral connotations. Upright citizens stand tall with their shoulders back. They're honest, honourable, upstanding, respectable, reputable, high-minded, law-abiding, right-minded, worthy, moral, ethical, righteous, decent, good, virtuous, principled, proper, just, noble, incorruptible, conscientious, and, importantly, CORRECT. And this moral discourse has influenced eating etiquette.

Eating for us humans is not just a way to transfer food to the stomach. In many cultures, there's an entire upright eating etiquette. Whereby manners maketh the man (or woman), and to avoid eating like a pig (or a quadruped), we must sit up straight or "correctly," without slouching or leaning back, never leaning on our elbows. We hold our cutlery "correctly" using specific techniques and, in particular, we bring our forks to our mouths, against gravity. Quadrupeds, of course, lower their heads to their food.

It is quite possible that, unwittingly, we have transposed this bipedal feeding etiquette to breastfeeding without ever taking into account that our babies are quadrupeds. These observations lead us to highlight a received idea that has perhaps regulated maternal breastfeeding posture since Egyptian times. It is quite possible that people have always thought that mothers should breastfeed using the same "correct" upright positions in which they themselves eat and why we have accepted holding our babies while struggling against gravity. And maybe that's also why Peiper characterised human babies as obligate dorsal feeders. Peiper just never saw human babies as quadrupeds.

Biological nurturing likely helps to resolve this mother–baby positional conflict. That's because BN enables full neonatal abdominal feeding positions together with comfortable, relaxing positions for the mother, using gravity positively for both. But the positional paradox affects how we introduce biological nurturing, or laid-back breastfeeding, to mothers.

Many health professionals have written to me saying that mothers don't want to lean back when they suggest they try BN. Mothers also write saying that a semi-reclined posture doesn't feel natural. As soon as I realised that this resistance may be associated with the bipedal need of *Homo sapiens* to be upright, including all the proper, correct, and ethical connotations, I changed the way I talked to mothers. I stopped suggesting that biological nurturing positions were natural because they aren't. Instead, I suggest that mothers get comfortable. No mother has ever refused comfort, but many will tell you that they are uncomfortable leaning back. Mothers often say it doesn't feel right or that they are losing control. And that's probably just because human mothers are bipedal, struggling to be upright citizens against gravity.

All living creatures are subjected to the forces of gravity. The taller we are, the greater the burden. From an evolutionary perspective, it makes sense that each species would have strategies aiding them to accomplish those activities that are necessary for survival. In the next chapter, we summarise the gravitational mechanisms that make biological nurturing work. Going with gravity not only helps mothers and babies get started with breastfeeding but it also appears to increase enjoyment.

CHAPTER 13

Going with Gravity

T he positive use of gravity is integral to the success of biological nurturing and influences two important mechanical factors. First, gravity promotes close mother–baby body apposition. And second, gravity smooths jerky reflex movements, promoting neonatal locomotion when the degree of maternal body slope is favourable. In turn, these factors appear to influence the synergy between BN postures and positions. Therefore, gravitational forces play a central role in the expression of primitive neonatal reflexes – either as stimulants or as barriers to successful breastfeeding.

The mechanisms have to do with gravitational drag exerting pressure, which draws the baby towards the centre of the earth. When a breastfeeding mother sits upright, gravity drags the baby straight down the maternal torso towards the pillow, the mother's lap, and the floor. The baby reflex movements, released through positional brushing, often appear jerky and uncoordinated. The more upright the mother, the greater the amplitude or breadth of those baby movements, such as hand-to-mouth, and arm and leg cycling, so often associated with breast fighting or latch refusal. The greater the breadth, the stronger the mother must grip her baby's back and neck to keep baby in place and at breast level.

In contrast, laid-back maternal sitting postures go with gravity. The direction of the centre of the earth shifts and that same gravitational drag pulls the baby through the mother's body, maintaining close body apposition and helping to keep him in place. Gravity also blunts the strength and amplitude of jerky reflex expression. Mothers no longer need to hold on tightly to the baby's back, neck or head, although mothers trying BN for the

Figure 35: Experimenting with BN

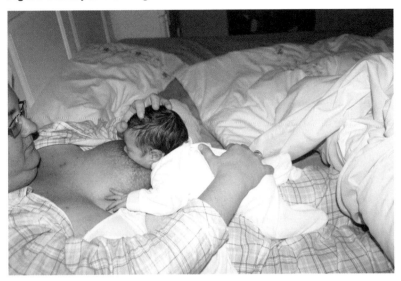

Janneke Hoek-Nijssen from the Netherlands uses this photo taken of her and baby Ismee to show mothers how to get started with biological nurturing.

first time often apply light pressure to support the baby's head (see Figure 35).

How Can the Milk Flow Up?

Some people have asked about milk flow in BN positions, wondering how the milk can flow upward to the baby, seemingly against gravity. Of course, this would not be a good position for bottle feeding. However, the breastfed baby extracts the milk aided by the milk-ejection reflex. Often, the milk-ejection reflex is very strong, and many babies have difficulty controlling the flow. A laid-back breastfeeding position helps with this. First, the strong flow is somewhat reduced by gravity. And second, the baby, with no pressure along his back, neck or head, controls the feed and often comes off spontaneously, waiting for the flow to calm.

Weight is another factor that influences the force of gravitational drag. The more the baby weighs, the greater the pull of gravity. This may be one explanation as to why some mothers who sit upright to breastfeed develop sore nipples after the first couple of days or weeks.

Parallel Angles on Birth and Breastfeeding

For over a quarter of a century there has been scientific evidence demonstrating how gravity affects labour and birth, and there is an interesting parallel between biological nurturing and the positional changes for birth that were proposed in the 1980s. Freedom of position is often restricted during labour. During active management, for example, the foetal heart rate must be assessed following surgical rupture of the membranes. Mothers usually sit semi-reclined in bed and are strapped to a monitor.

A prime index of progress in labour is the descent of the foetal head. Optimally, with each contraction, pressure is applied evenly down the foetal axis, reaching the presenting part (usually the vertex of the flexed foetal head). This pressure aids cervical dilatation. An upright or all fours position works with gravity, promoting foetal descent and opening the cervix. When mothers are recumbent, semi-recumbent, or sitting in bed, labour contractions may be less effective as they must work against gravity. During labour, these laid-back maternal positions close the pelvis, exerting constant sacral pressure, making the ischial-sacral and coccyx joints immobile and, as a result, often delay the descent of the foetal head.

Nevertheless, obstetricians and midwives traditionally encouraged mothers to give birth lying on their sides, in a semi-Fowler's position, or with their feet in stirrups in a lithotomy position. American midwife Ina May Gaskin, anthropologist Sheila Kitzinger, childbirth educator Janet Balaskas, and French obstetrician Michel Odent suggested in the 1980s that being upright during labour and birth has mechanical advantages, using gravity positively. Although freedom of position during labour and birth immediately resonated with many mothers, many health professionals remained unconvinced, leading to heated debate. Today in the UK, it is recognised that the positive use of gravity reduces the need for pharmaceutical pain relief and helps to keep birth "normal."

Likewise, the "laid-back" breastfeeding posture, the BN component enabling the positive use of gravity, also challenges our beliefs about the best position to use when breastfeeding, sometimes creating heated discussion. Many mothers immediately embraced the concept, but a number of British health practitioners have remained sceptical.

In both instances, the postures suggested for centuries as "correct" to achieve a reproductive outcome did not take into account gravitational forces. There is a certain irony in that our assumptions about the correct positions for birth work for breastfeeding and those for breastfeeding work for birth. Our beliefs and convictions have been turned on their head – by gravity!

Like gravity, neonatal sleep states also mitigate the strength and amplitude of reflex expression, helping to smooth and soften erratic reflex movements. In the next chapter, we turn our attention to the impact of neonatal behavioural state upon breastfeeding initiation.

CHAPTER 14

Neonatal Behavioural State

Everyone knows that babies sleep abundantly – almost all the time. But what does this mean? How do we define sleep? What is the nature and quality of foetal versus neonatal sleep? Importantly, what is the optimal sleep environment? These questions motivated doctors like Wolff in the 1950s, and André-Thomas, Prechtl, and Brazelton in the 1960s to examine sleep versus awake states of neonatal consciousness. This differentiation was vital to the development of reliability in neurological assessment. Indeed, Brazelton recounts his light-bulb moment when he realised that neonatal behavioural state is "the critical matrix on which to base all other neonatal reactions – sensory as well as motor".[1]

Simply put, behavioural state is the level of arousal ranging from deep sleep to crying states. Initially, an electroencephalogram (EEG) was necessary to define neonatal behavioural state. However, Brazelton described observable neonatal behaviours that regularly occur together during EEG observations, characterising sleep and awake states. Brazelton's work eliminated the need for an EEG to define the baby's state. Instead, he produced valid definitions based solely upon behavioural observations of movement (eye, facial, and body), heart and respiratory rate, and vocalizations.[2]

In Chapter 4, we introduced important links between foetal and neonatal sleep states and, in particular, light or REM sleep. Active or light sleep is characterised by rapid-eye movement (REM) and has been termed "wide-awake sleep." REM sleep is associated with learning because brain activity is similar to brainwaves in awake states. Babies, like adults, process information that is entered into memory. Sleep patterns change as the central nervous system (CNS) develops but motor activity occurs during sleep and awake states in both foetus and neonate. [3] Let us now look again in greater depth at the evidence explaining how babies' sleep patterns progress from womb to world.

Foetal Life

Sleep-wake behavioural states, with patterns of organised cycles of rest and movement, develop at approximately 32 gestational weeks. Foetal behavioural states are determined by heart rate, presence or absence of REM, and body movements. REM sleep develops from 28 to 30 gestational weeks, whereas deep sleep only develops much later (around 36 gestational weeks). The foetus transitions so rapidly from state to state that most of the time the baby is in "indeterminate," transitional sleep, which lacks clear definition.[4,5] The foetal sleep cycle consists of changes from REM sleep to awake states and lasts about 40 minutes.[6-8]

Neonatal Life

At birth, the newborn also sleeps for up to 18 hours a day. But neonatal sleep is neither fully diurnal nor does it follow a light/dark pattern. The brand newborn sleep cycle lasts approximately the same amount of time as the foetal cycle (from 20 to 50 minutes). This is approximately half the length of the adult sleep cycle (90 minutes). Newborns spend half their total sleep time in REM sleep. However, indeterminate sleep continues to dominate for at least the first 6 to 8 postnatal weeks as the CNS matures.

Neonatal sleep function continues to mature throughout the first year, increasing the duration of deep sleep and decreasing periods of light REM or active sleep with a greater number of full sleep cycles occurring consecutively. This lengthens nap times and extends the duration of night-time sleep.[9-11] Taken together, this evidence suggests that increased sleep duration is a natural part of growth and development, not reliant on method of feeding or resulting from sleep training techniques.

Doctoral Research: State Definitions and Results

For my PhD research, I modelled my operational definitions upon Brazelton's six neonatal behavioural states. However, I changed "fussy" to "agitated" and identified three sleep and three awake states, whereas traditionally, a drowsy state (between asleep and awake) is usually called an awake state. Therefore, the three sleep states were deep, light (REM), and drowsy, and the awake states were quiet alert, agitated, and crying.

Paediatricians usually carry out reflex evaluation when babies are awake to enhance reliability. This is because sleep states are known to either suppress the expression of primitive neonatal reflexes (PNRs) or blunt their strength and amplitude. My findings demonstrated that only two of the 20 PNRs, leg cycling and crawling, were not observed in the sleep states.

As soon as I had this raw data, I experienced my own light-bulb moment. Compelling BN video clips illustrated how almost half my breastfeeding sample (*n*=19) latched on in either light-REM sleep (*n*=9) or drowsy (*n*=10) states. During milk transfer, more babies were sleeping (*n*=25) than awake, ticking all the boxes indicating excellent milk transfer. At latch, babies were, for the most part, in indeterminate sleep. That is, they moved rapidly from light-REM to drowsy sleep states and back again. Importantly, these results confirmed that early breast attachment and active suckling are simple reflex behaviours, not intentional. Intention implies thought. Intention is a plan and linked to the will to act, which can only occur when you're awake.

Traditional Advice

Mothers often ask: "When or how often should I feed my baby?" Kathryn Barnard, an American nurse with a passion for early mother–baby interactions, was a founder of the Nursing Child Assessment Satellite Training (NCAST).[12] She created a chart offering guidance for mothers and nurses. I have summarised this advice that health professionals have traditionally given to mothers for four of the behavioural states in Figure 36.

These recommendations continue to underpin our infant feeding policies and you can see that mothers are advised to wait until babies are awake and cue that they are ready to feed. The quiet alert state is said to be optimal.[13–20]

Barnard was highly influenced by Brazelton's innovation suggesting that behavioural state is the critical matrix, a bedrock for neonatal activity. This literally changed the nurses' work ethic, transforming the organization of the baby's day in special and intensive care units. Nurses prioritised sleep over procedures. Babies were no longer awakened for X-rays, ultrasound, and heel pricks. Instead, nurses went on baby time. Understandably, they would never attempt to feed a sleeping baby.

However, Barnard's feeding recommendations also mirror our cultural assumptions and expectations of sleep and eating patterns. In our industrialised nations, sleep has a sacred status. Everybody knows that sleep is restorative. We sleep in bed alone or with our partners, isolated from the world, protecting deep sleep. Based upon our own needs, we assume that babies require a

Figure 36: Old-School Feeding Advice (which often delays breast-feeding initiation)

Deep Sleep	Light REM Sleep
Any attempts to feed will be frustrating. Babies will be unresponsive. Wait to feed until baby transitions to a more responsive state. Do not attempt to feed. 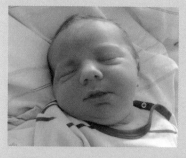	Baby is not yet ready to feed even if he makes brief fussy or crying sounds. Baby is not alert enough to feed. 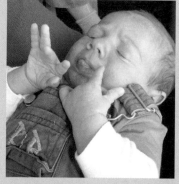
Drowsy	**Quiet Alert**
Wait to see if baby will return to sleep. Left alone and without stimuli, baby may go back to sleep. To wake baby up, give him something to suck as this may arouse him to a quiet alert state. 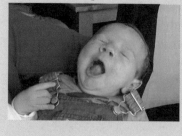	This is the ideal state to feed the baby providing much pleasure and positive feedback for mother. It is an excellent time to initiate BF before baby becomes fussy and agitated. 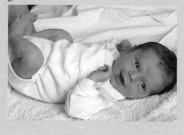

designated place and should be left alone, undisturbed, in a cot.

In addition, we think that babies only feed in awake states based on our own eating habits. Most mothers associate feeding with waking the baby and usually pick their baby up in response to a baby hunger cue, such as crying. Crying is accepted culturally as the normal verbal way for a baby to indicate hunger. However, from a human needs perspective, crying for food indicates that your most basic needs are not being met. Imagine if adults had to burst into tears to indicate that they were ready for dinner every evening.

Behavioural State Breastfeeding Mechanisms

By contrast, in my research, I encouraged mothers to put their sleeping babies to the breast. In Chapter 4, we discussed how navel radiation and movement are released in the womb while the foetus sleeps. Once babies are born, sleep states do not inhibit navel radiation. Rather, they enhance this to and fro movement. The stimulation from constant close ventral contact in BN positions is vital to trigger the body brushing that releases PNR locomotion. Latching and breastfeeding happen spontaneously.

Importantly, consistent with paediatric findings, the strength of PNR response at the breast is diminished in sleep states. For physicians evaluating the integrity of the baby's nervous system, sleep states were a drawback reducing reliability of assessment. However, in the breastfeeding context, this is advantageous. As soon as they're born, babies transition rapidly into agitated and crying states. The more agitated the baby, the more erratic the reflexes, the more difficult it is to latch. Like gravity, sleep smooths irregular and jerky reflex movements. Latching in sleep states actually helps.

That explains why my PhD results suggest that feeding babies in sleep states reduces breast boxing and latch refusal. Those behaviours, often characterised by jerky cogwheel movements, often thwart latch when mothers wait for the baby to cue and sit upright to breastfeed.

The BN value system places great importance upon keeping the baby in his natural habitat during the first 48 to 72 hours. We cannot say it often enough: this address is cheek to breast when the baby's sleeping. While sleeping, babies cue in various ways. Maternal response is quicker because mothers often recognise the cues spontaneously in a tactile instead of a visual way. This is not surprising. In BN, babies are on their mothers' bodies. The movements are familiar. This evidence challenges the well-documented belief that "a sleeping baby will not feed, and a hungry baby will not sleep." This also calls into question the necessity of any newborn baby, in our industrialised world, having to cue by crying for a feed.

What Are Feeding Cues?

Feeding cues are simple inborn reflex movements that aid babies to find the breast and latch. In the first days, they are involuntary. In other words, the baby does not intend or plan to cue but the spontaneous movement in itself triggers latch. The cueing reflexes are released by internal or external stimuli. A low blood sugar, hunger, a mother's touch, body brushing or contact with thin air all release feeding cues. See Table 5 for a list of some reflex feeding cues.

Feeding cues are not behavioural states, although crying is both a cue and a state (because crying is a vocalization). In other words, when the baby moves his eyes rapidly under closed eyelids, this is not a feeding cue. Rapid eye movement is one of many behaviours that regularly occur together, characterising light sleep. Random movement, irregular breathing, smiles or grimaces, brief fussy sounds and delayed reaction to light, sound or touch are other valid indicators of REM sleep. The baby may transition from light sleep to a drowsy state or return to a deep sleep state. What is new is that light or REM sleep is an ideal state in which to initiate breastfeeding. Figure 37 summarises neonatal behavioural state, illustrating the BN perspective.

Table 5: Baby-Feeding Reflex Cues

Hand-to-mouth
Mouth gape
Tongue-dart or licking the breast
Arm–leg cycle
Finger extension, flexion
Lip smacking
Sucking movements
Horizontal rooting
Vertical head bobbing
Cardinal reflex – lip movements

If a Baby's Not Cueing for a Feed, Why Put Him to Breast?

The simple answer to that question is because in BN positions, sleeping babies latch on and feed and this can be particularly helpful during the time of initiation. But let us now examine some scientific reasons.

The first concerns the rapidity of newborn state transitions. Brazelton and Nugent outline procedures in the Neonatal Behavioural Assessment Scale (NBAS) .[21] If a baby maintains an active alert state for 30 seconds during his third day evaluation, he obtains a high score demonstrating developmental maturation. Newborn babies change state so rapidly that during the time it takes to carry out the NBAS evaluation (15–20 minutes), the baby can change state up to 24 times.[22,23]

Unfortunately, when baby is in a cot, the state transitions can be so rapid that by the time the mother sees the cue, picks the baby up, adjusts her clothes, finds the pillow, and finally puts baby to breast, many have transitioned into a crying state or back into deeper sleep.

Second, as stated above, deep sleep is anabolic, promoting growth and development. Having a number of full sleep cycles during a nap is restorative. However, the newborn baby's needs are not satisfied in the same way as an adult. For us, being isolated in our familiar, quiet, dark room is usually the right address. We feel safe and protected from environmental disturbances. This leads to a repeated number of full sleep cycles. But suppose you were returning home from an exhausting day's work and you fell asleep on the bus traveling from the airport to your home, an hour's distance away. Suppose the bus driver failed to notice you asleep as he parked in the depot. You would surely awaken to find yourself sitting alone in the dark, in the middle of nowhere on a bus parked for the night: a very frightening experience!

Likewise, although the distances are not the same, mothers often say that each time they put the baby in the cot, instead of settling he wakes up. Just like you feel protected in your bed, with the familiar smells and surroundings, when you BN a sleeping baby, you protect the integrity of the sleep cycle and increase the opportunity to have repeated sleep cycles. This happens because the maternal body nest is a familiar place. Mothers spontaneously reduce any effects from environmental disturbances that might wake the baby.

Third, and importantly, a repeated number of sleep cycles increases the number of indeterminate transitional sleep episodes. It is precisely during these transitions that babies often latch on and breastfeed. As discussed previously, early and frequent latchments imprint the baby to the breast and increase feeding frequency. Babies accomplish metabolic adaptation sooner.

Furthermore, we know that light REM sleep aids memory. More latchments transitioning to or from REM light sleep subconsciously help the baby recall and memorise his individual suckling patterns. Feeding reflexes become conditioned sooner. During the first weeks, the repetition of these

Figure 37: Neonatal Behavioural States

	Deep Sleep	Light Sleep	Drowsy
Description	Quiet sleep, sound asleep, heavy sleep, fast asleep.	REM sleep, paradox or wide awake sleep.	Dozing; half asleep, half awake, twilight sleep, dazed.
Body Activity	Still, occasional startle or jerk	Some random movement but low activity; may make rooting, sucking movements	Variable, mild startles; Smooth gross movement. Little overall motor activity
Eyes	Closed, no movement	Closed; rapid eye movements (REM) under closed lids	Flutter, when open are heavy lidded, dull gazed
Breathing	Deep, smooth, regular may snore.	Irregular.	Irregular.
Face	Occasional sucking.	May smile or grimace. Brief vocalisations.	Still, may smile, grimace, suck, or tongue dart.
Level of Response	Resistant to any stimulation; slight reaction when repeated then blocks out sound light & touch.	Delayed response to light, sound & touch, may return to deep sleep or arouse to drowsy.	Reactive but delayed; if stimulated repeatedly will awaken.
Feeding advice	Practise BN cheek to breast for as long as mother wants. If problems, encourage mum to BN sleeping baby for 1 hour.	Although delayed response, newborn often latches; aiding mother & baby to discover what works during first weeks; optimises learning & memory.	Babies root & latch; ideal feeding state whenever there are problems (latching, sore nipples, engorgement).

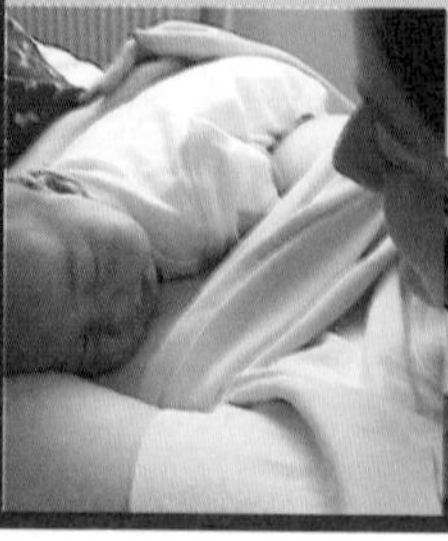

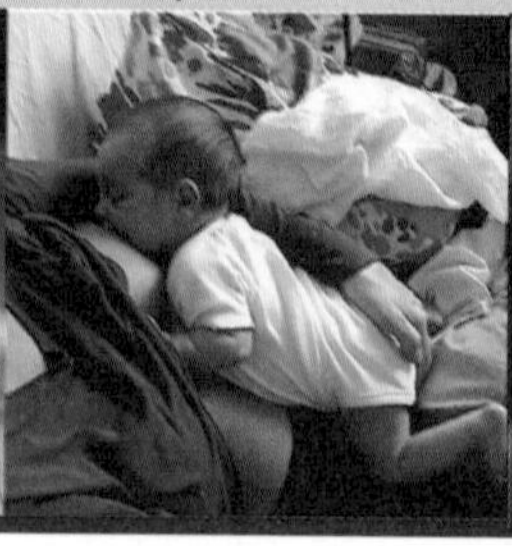

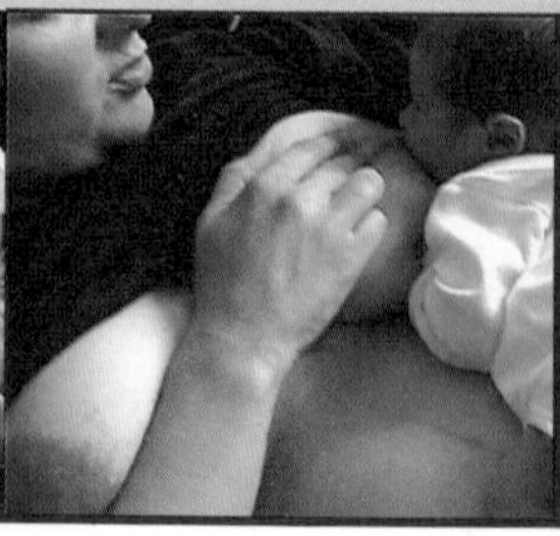

Quiet Alert	Agitated	Crying
Awake, alert, quiet or active alert, focused & communicative.	Loss of focus; may fuss = audible sound <1 minute; may have worried look.	Loud vocalisation lasting >1 minute.
Limited motion, minimum motor activity, may track sound involving head movement.	Increased motor activity, arm & leg cycles may posit or hiccup.	High motor activity; arm thrashing, leg flailing, back arching sometimes stiffening.
Open, may track objects	When open, may appear hyper alert; sometimes closed	Open or tightly closed.
Regular.	Irregular.	Fast & irregular with possible short periods of apnea.
Few movements; has bright-eyed look with invested focus on stimulus, may coo.	Grimace, pucker, frown; mouth opening, tongue extrusion, often no sound; colour may flush.	Mouth gape, tongue curl, audible loud cry, skin colour flushed may become ruddy.
Concentrated, focused, attention to stimuli	Losing control but may respond to words; hypersensitive as becomes overly responsive to stimuli.	Reactive, out of control, extreme response to external/internal stimuli.
Ideal feeding state unless there are any problems; Once BF is established, optimal state to initiate BF.	Often difficult to initiate BF. Mum may need to calm baby before BF unless baby can latch quickly & easily.	Mum will need to console baby before BF unless baby latches immediately.

143

early patterns is how feeding reflexes become intentional.

We have introduced many baby benefits but breastfeeding the sleeping baby also benefits mothers because they have more time, in a calm environment, to discover what works. Read one mother's testimony below.

◆

TESTIMONIAL

I have struggled with breastfeeding partially due to lack of milk. At 10 weeks, I finally got my daughter to nurse a little, but she still often refuses the breast in favour of bottle. I have started to figure out how to catch her just as she is waking up and get her to latch on before she is fully awake. I felt like I was tricking her but after watching the video clip on the biological nurturing internet site, I wonder if this is just natural.

I wish I had seen this when I was pregnant. If I had understood what you are teaching, I think things would have been very different in the first days of my daughter's life.

◆

Reflection

It's not just latch that would have been easier for this mother. It's quite likely that the only reason she thought that she had insufficient milk was because every time her daughter breastfed herself to sleep, she put her in the cot. After a few minutes, typically she awakened and cried. Her interpretation, like millions of other mothers, was that she didn't have enough milk.

Does All This Mean That Mothers Should Sleep with Their Babies?

Not necessarily, but that discussion exceeds the scope of this book. However, the BN perspective is clear: mothers should hold their sleeping babies for as often and as long as they want. But in doing so, if mothers feel irresistibly sleepy, then they should put their babies "back to sleep" in a safe place. This is because babies and children always require a designated responsible person who is awake to nurture and protect them. The UK BFI presents a balanced approach in their excellent nighttime guidelines for parents and for health professionals, including guidelines for safe bedsharing. They state a principal that underpins all breastfeeding support: "it isn't helpful to tell parents what they must or mustn't do; instead, listen carefully and offer information appropriate to their needs".[24,25] Importantly, everyone in the family needs to have enough sleep and to sleep safely. The aim is to inform parents objectively about research so that they can make informed decisions.

Implications for Practice

Many mothers are left feeling confused by the quality and quantity of sleep necessary to promote their baby's well-being during the first weeks. Few health professionals, however, discuss neonatal behavioural state with pregnant mothers. Mothers lack information about the immaturity of deep sleep function. No one mentions that many babies experience difficulty transitioning into deep sleep or back into fully awake states. Mothers are often unaware of the rapid state changes and the resulting abrupt and fluctuating sleep patterns.

Doing BN with the sleeping baby at the right address during the first postnatal weeks is a way for mothers to assess their baby's individual sleep patterns. Mothers protect baby's sleep, temperature, and breathing all at the same time. In that way they get to know their baby's rhythms and needs more quickly. Because the neonatal sleep cycle is so short, and the capacity for deep sleep so immature, many babies do not sleep well on their own during the first postnatal year. In the first weeks, doing BN when baby is in sleep states may help to develop smooth transitions and to keep babies in deep sleep for longer. It also helps mothers overcome those initial glitches or difficulties often associated with breastfeeding initiation, such as fighting the breast, baby too sleepy to latch, engorgement, and sore nipples.

Health professionals should also inform mothers that babies who are held and carried cry less, conserving both maternal and neonatal energy, as well as increasing the maternal enjoyment that should go hand in hand with having a new baby. Once breastfeeding feels established, some mothers will opt to continue to carry the baby using a sling, even around the house. This is sometimes called babywearing and many mothers find this beneficial.[26]

However, such parenting styles are countercultural in our industrialised society, and many well-intentioned but misinformed people firmly believe that mothers must keep their newborn babies in a cot between breastfeeds during the early days. It has been almost 50 years since Montagu, the famous anthropologist, suggested that a period of external gestation is beneficial.[27] Health professionals can help by sharing this message with mothers, and supporting and reassuring those who would choose to keep their babies close.

CHAPTER 15

Maternal Hormonal State

Brazelton's work examining baby's behavioural state was inspiring. I took the Neonatal Behavioral Assessment Scale (NBAS) training and started to observe, describe, and group objectively the baby's actions, reactions, and clinical features. Soon, I found that I could identify the baby's behavioural state at a glance. Then suddenly, in another light-bulb moment, I realised that, unconsciously, I was also observing the mother's behaviours. By observing her actions – the things she said and did, her body tone, movements, and colouring – I started to notice patterns. Mothers' faces, eyes, gaze, mouth, and complexion were particularly revealing and could change radically.

When mothers sat upright, in skin-to-skin contact or lightly dressed, they often appeared alert with eyes wide open, concentrating, trying to remember the instructions they had received to obtain the "correct" latch. They kept looking at me for guidance and support. Their vocalisations were often complaints. They said: "I can't get baby to open his mouth wide enough." "I just can't get her to latch." "I just don't have enough hands to breastfeed!"

Mothers sitting bolt upright often had tense and unbalanced shoulders. The side holding the baby was often raised awkwardly. Her wrist was often at right angles to her forearm, bearing all the weight of the baby. When sitting upright, mothers who were experiencing problems were often pale and tense. They often had constricted facial expressions with a furrowed brow and a brooding or worried look.

Just looking at these mothers could make me feel uneasy and I would place pillows around them to support their bodies, trying to make them more comfortable. This usually resulted in an immediate change in maternal posture. Moving from ischial to sacral sitting is a backward rocking motion. Mothers sat semi-reclined without realising it and gazed at their babies. Now their backs were leaning against the chair, bed, or sofa.

When babies were asleep, mothers' eyes immediately softened; when babies were awake, they established eye-to-eye contact and often started to coo. Behavioural changes were accompanied by visible physical relaxation. Mothers' shoulders dropped, and they seemed to melt into the comfort of body support. Their eyes closed and then gently opened with a glazed look. Mothers' eyes often remained half-closed as though they were shutting out the world: their jaws went slack, mouths opened in a half-smile, and it was not long before a facial glow or flush appeared. But the most striking change was a complete focus upon the baby.

Initially, it was unclear how or why this happened. Was relaxation the result or the releaser of this change? Or did it have something to do with the baby?

Curiously, for the mothers who perceived they had breastfeeding problems, these behavioural changes did not occur immediately. They carried on looking at me with a worried expression. So I found myself describing the baby to focus their gaze. I said things like, "Wow! Did your baby just smile?" or "The baby's eyelashes are so long…" or "I've never seen a newborn baby with that much hair!." The mother then looked at her baby and it was like she discovered her baby for the first time. Their intimacy quickly excluded all external interactions.

As said previously, worry and anxiety are the enemies of reproductive events, such as pregnancy, birth, and breastfeeding. I tried to mimic the way I support mothers in labour. I do not engage them in everyday conversation, ask them questions, or tell them what to do. My mission is to get them to focus on the baby. When they are with their babies, instead of with me, daily events, fear, or anxiety, the contractions are usually strong and regular. The birth is usually spontaneous. These mechanisms were easy to transfer to the breastfeeding context.

In the first 48 hours, few breastfeeding mothers have problems, but they are often somewhat anxious or worried about getting started. During the hospital stay, usually all that midwives need do is to get mothers to comfortably gaze at their babies. BN maternal postures ensure that mothers gaze at their babies without craning their necks. In turn, just looking at the baby often releases a cascade of instinctual mothering behaviours. We know that looking at or thinking about the baby releases oxytocin and I interpreted these behaviours as being associated with high levels of oxytocin pulsatility.

The Role of Oxytocin

Oxytocin, a peptide hormone, is well known for its contraction and ejection effects. Produced in the hypothalamus and stored in the posterior pituitary gland, oxytocin is not released in a steady stream but rather in pulses; and high peaks of pulsatility are associated with orgasm, ejaculation, foetus ejection, and milk release.[1] The contraction/ejection effects are often termed mechanical or peripheral because they can be caused to occur artificially through the intravenous infusion of synthetic oxytocin (trademarked Syntocinon or Pitocin).

The synthetic form is often used to contract the uterus to augment labour or mixed with ergometrine to control postpartum bleeding. The synthetic molecule is too large to cross the blood–brain barrier and therefore Pitocin or Syntocinon remain peripheral, achieving good contraction and ejection effect but not impregnating the brain.[2]

I remember presenting my preliminary research results at a Royal Society of Medicine breastfeeding conference in 2002. My interpretations, related to the behavioural effects of oxytocin, were completely ignored. Today, there is an increasing body of good quality research evidence suggesting that oxytocin has central or behavioural effects, which only occur when it is released into the bloodstream directly by the brain, the effects of which, many studies have suggested, promote social, sexual, and maternal behaviours.[3,4,5]

Importantly, although oxytocin has always been recognised as the contraction/ejection hormone in the reproductive lives of men and women, it also plays an important role in everyday life. Occasionally, sharing a meal with loved ones, for example, will likely promote high levels of oxytocin under certain conditions. Many parents will recognise that this can happen unexpectedly, maybe at dusk, over dinner. Children can suddenly become attentive and interested in what's being said, listening to each other, and replying with understanding and affection. You may suddenly feel overcome with love for them and they for you. It doesn't happen often but when it does, it's almost spiritual.

It's the same feeling you can have if you sing in a choir. Oxytocin is probably the hormone that underpins that overwhelming feeling of unity when everyone starts singing with one voice. That is why so many people now call oxytocin the "love/cuddle hormone." This is also why Kerstin Uvnäs Moberg, the world recognised leader in oxytocin research, wrote a book in 2013 entitled *The Hormone of Closeness: The Role of Oxytocin in Relationships.*[6]

It is well known that an environment conducive to high oxytocin pulsatility, in hospital or at home, is associated with normal vaginal birth without any need for intervention. However, the potential effects of maintaining high maternal concentrations from pregnancy to birth to breastfeeding and into the early postnatal weeks are less well known. Results from research carried out by Uvnäs Moberg and her team from Sweden suggest that this may be important. For example:

- Maternal oxytocin concentrations are higher immediately following birth than at any time during labour.[7]
- Higher maternal oxytocin pulsatility on the second postnatal day is associated with increased breastfeeding duration at 6 weeks.[8]
- Oxytocin has an anti stress effect. Each suckling episode is followed by a decrease in blood pressure and breastfeeding mothers are calmer. This correlates with oxytocin concentrations.[9,10]

See Figure 38 to compare observations of physiological and behavioural features from birth to breastfeeding that appear to indicate high maternal pulsatility. If I apply their findings to my clinical work, if I can just get a mother to look like this on the second postnatal day, she will likely be more relaxed and breastfeed for six weeks.

Observations of mothers who are transported by events are supported by some research evidence suggesting that oxytocin induces states of euphoria and forgetfulness.[11] Marsha Walker, an American nurse and IBCLC, states

Figure 38: Behavioural Continuity from Birth to Breastfeeding

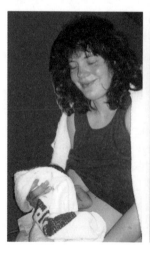
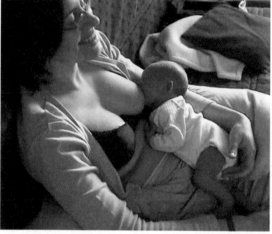

that uterine contractions, sometimes called "afterpains," experienced during breastfeeding are also indicators of successful milk transfer, although this kind of observation only reflects the mechanical effects of high oxytocin concentrations.[12] Building upon Walker's comments, close, but discreet, observations of the mothers in my study revealed erect nipples that could also be interpreted as mechanical indicators. Increased thirst is yet another index that research suggests is associated with high oxytocin pulsatility, and it is well known that breastfeeding mothers increase their fluid intake.[13]

Just as clusters of features define neonatal behavioural states, theoretically it was possible that these observations could be viewed as part of a hormonal profile supporting lactation. I introduced new terminology to describe these emerging behavioural patterns suggestive of high maternal oxytocin pulsatility. Instead of using Brazelton's model and saying a "maternal behavioural state indicative of high oxytocin pulsatility," I used an umbrella term, *hormonal complexion*. Table 6 summarises the behavioural clusters that I suggest are indicators of a maternal oxytocin complexion.

We continue to discuss and refine these characteristics within expert groups that supported the doctoral work, and among health professionals and others who are certified BN Breastfeeding Companions. Today, "hormonal complexion" is being developed as a theoretical construct and the hormonal theory supporting these observations is summarised below.

Developing Theory

It is not unusual to associate colours with emotions and physical states of being: green with envy, red with anger or heat or a flush of excitement, and blue with melancholy. Similarly, stress, frustration, fear, and fight-or-flight behaviours (especially where reaction is inhibited) can be observed as biochemical responses in people's facial expressions suggesting, for example, a cortisol or an adrenalin complexion.

Importantly, Uvnäs Moberg highlights that oxytocin is a shy hormone and her assessment personifies my clinical experience. An oxytocin hormonal complexion often feels bashful in the company of loud, nervous, worried people who ask many questions or who make negative comments. Oxytocin pulsatility also runs away from people who observe, or peer, prod, or touch. For example, performing a vaginal examination during labour often makes mothers' contractions stop. People who teach or guide or show mothers how to breastfeed, for example, will inevitably diminish high oxytocin pulsatility. Furthermore, oxytocin pulsatility dislikes cold, bright light, and other brash environments. There's a strong argument that endogenous oxytocin is in

Table 6: Colson's Clusters: Characteristics of an Oxytocin Hormonal Complexion

Oxytocin: Behavioural Effects	Oxytocin: Mechanical Effects
Eyes partially closed, may be glazed.	Nipple erect at latch.
May gaze at sleeping baby or establish intimate eye-to-eye contact. May look into space.	Opposite nipple moist, pearling or leaking.
Euphoric expression.	Age-appropriate afterpains.
Half-smile.	Gush of lochia during feeding.
Facial glow or blush.	Thirst.
Unresponsive to questions; if vocalises, sentences often remain unfinished.	
Forgetful.	
Drowsy.	
Low body tone.	
Slow regular breathing.	
Absence of shoulder hunching or tension.	
Slack jaw.	

Table 7: Threats to High Oxytocin Pulsatility

Bright lights, cold temperature.
Looking closely, peering or staring at mothers.
Explaining procedures with furrowed brow and/or establishing close, direct eye-to-eye contact.
Teaching, Guiding, Giving directions.
Thinking prompted by asking questions, mundane conversation.
Fear.
Pain.
Discomfort.
Worry, Anxiety.

Maternal Hormonal Complexion: A Theory [14]

We have said previously that changing from upright to laid-back postures often induces a state of relaxation and what we have described as an oxytocic maternal complexion.

Breastfeeding mothers were observed to alter their behaviours during episodes of BN. These changes seemed to coincide with a physical shift from reliance upon ischial sitting to sacral sitting. The before/after BN observations from the videotapes were so striking that we started thinking about possible explanations and a physiological mechanism for these behavioural changes slowly emerged. As mothers changed from upright to laid-back postures, the movements of sacral nutation and counter-nutation occurred.

Physiologically, this movement, well recognised by cranial osteopaths, could travel up the spinal column to release a burst of oxytocin, which, we can recall, is stored in the posterior pituitary gland. Therefore, it is possible that central release of oxytocin could be influenced by complex systems of sacral/occipital miming actions. Simply put, through flexion of the sacrum, a mother could, theoretically, be stimulating her pituitary gland.

We acknowledge that the potential mechanism proposed for this phenomenon is purely speculative as no blood samples to measure maternal oxytocin concentrations were taken to give any physiological credence to these interpretations. However, these compelling visual data build upon the increasing amount of well-designed research carried out by Kerstin Uvnäs Moberg and her colleagues in Sweden, examining oxytocin and its behavioural effects, where blood samples were taken. Biological nurturing may be an intervention increasing oxytocin pulsatility as a bridging hormone from pregnancy to lactation. Further research is clearly required.

Video 7: Asking a question disturbs the flow of oxytocin

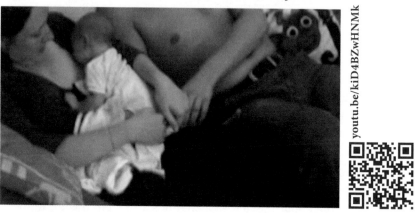

youtu.be/kiD4BZwHNMk

This clip illustrates pure family enjoyment as baby head bobs locating the nipple and attaching. I do not know what prompts me to ask them an unnecessary question as I am filming. Maybe because it looks like such fun. But all of a sudden, I ask them: "Do you do that often?" And with that, I completely break the mood.

short supply on most labour and postnatal wards. Table 7 illustrates and lists some common threats to oxytocin pulsatility.

It takes quite a while to learn how to adopt a "laid-back" approach when you work in a hospital on a busy labour or postnatal ward. I share with you a video clip of me filming a couple who are enjoying a lovely breastfeeding oxytocin moment. You will see the intimacy of the episode.

It's a great clip and I use it in all my BN certification workshops to illustrate how one innocent question can immediately destroy an oxytocin hormonal complexion.

The theory here suggests that an oxytocin hormonal complexion goes hand in hand with the expression of the innate maternal behaviours I observed, such as nesting, greeting, olfactory, transportation, grooming, body placing, gaze, and imitation. Compelling BN video data clearly suggest that human mothers have a species-specific innate instinctual behavioural capacity to breastfeed. And that is the subject of the next chapter.

CHAPTER 16

Instinctual Breastfeeding

Instinctual maternal behaviours are a key component of biological nurturing. The intervention is mother-centred. So often, interest showered upon the mother during pregnancy can be perceived as foetal attention: the mother is the vessel carrying the baby.[1] As soon as the baby is born, some argue that all interest in the mother ends. Entire books are written about the amazing newborn. How many books do you know that are entitled the amazing mother? Observe how maternal–infant reciprocity unfolds in Figure 39.

Practising biological nurturing, mothers take the lead. The baby is normally the only instruction book needed. My work suggests that mothers are truly amazing. Our research observations suggest that, in certain situations while sitting comfortably, gazing at the baby, mothers instinctively know how and when to release their baby's reflexes.

In contrast, using current approaches to breastfeeding initiation, mothers often think they will fail at breastfeeding even before they start! We use phrases like "attempting" or "trying to breastfeed." When mothers ask questions, instead of sharing our confidence in the unique biological design of a mother's body to nourish and nurture her baby, health professionals often suggest metaphors, saying that breastfeeding is like typing, riding a bike, dancing, or driving a car. These metaphors are not entirely accurate. These types of activities are learned skills and/or enhancements to increase enjoyment of life or to get ahead professionally, but they are not life-sustaining.

Breastfeeding your baby, on the other hand, lays the foundations for a lifelong relationship. Suckling is comparable to those activities of daily living

Figure 39: The Language of Discovery

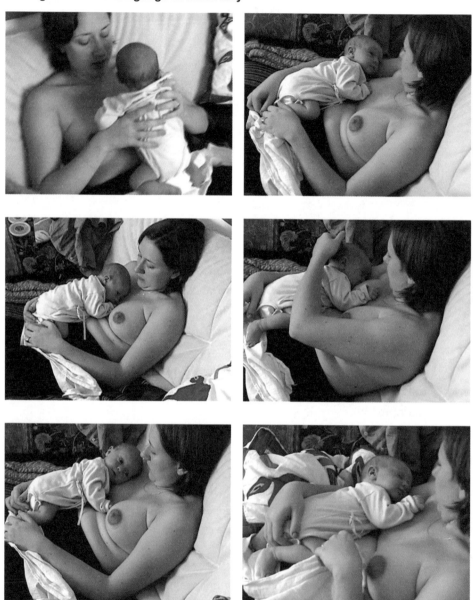

Biological nurturing is instinctive breastfeeding. When the mother's angle of recline enables comfortable baby gazing and/or eye-to-eye contact, mothers and babies converse spontaneously in a language of self discovery. Soft whispers, gentle stroking and grooming elicit baby's inborn feeding reflexes. In a veil of privacy, mothers' arms define the boundaries protecting the limits of her body nest. Bound in an intimate gaze they revel in the complicity of latch and satiety.

as defined in Roper, Logan, and Tierney's model of nursing.[2] Breastfeeding, in itself, maintains a safe environment and is an activity that is associated with breathing, communication, personal hygiene, mobility, eating, drinking, and expressing sexuality, among others.[3] The suggestion that breastfeeding is similar to learned activities often creates a "helpless" mother, dependent upon advice from experts at the very time when new mothers feel most vulnerable.

Biologically, and in countries untouched by lactation management, breastfeeding remains an activity of daily living for an average of four years for both mother and baby. There is mutual dependency when it is supposed to happen, at just the right time in the lifespan. Breastfeeding is certainly not something that the baby does by himself.

The word relationship implies, by definition, the give and take of two people. Mothers are active breastfeeders! They guide and protect their babies, aiding latch as necessary, through what we have observed as "emerging patterns of maternal instinctual behaviours".[4] Furthermore, mothers' participation is essential. Human mothers do not lie inert, rather they elicit or reply. Like any relationship, reciprocity enhances innate behavioural patterns, creating mother–child ties based upon love and respect. Mothers know more about their babies than anyone. They constantly assess their babies' well-being, detecting as soon as possible any deviation from the normal or potential problems.

The breastfeeding relationship, like any relationship, comprises both innate and acquired behaviours. However, for over a century, *breastfeeding as an acquired skill* – or the nurturing public health approach – has dominated our understanding and informed practice about how mothers best initiate breastfeeding. Biological nurturing restores the balance, bringing the nature or the instinctual component back into breastfeeding. Look at Figure 40.

This figure illustrates one such universal behaviour observed across the sample. When mothers and fathers are in positions of relaxation with their babies on top of their bodies, variations of the position called ventral suspension can be observed. I termed this spontaneous instinctual response "body placing."

Let us recall that ventral suspension concerns holding the baby around the thorax and is one of three positions used by paediatricians to release primitive neonatal reflexes, like placing, walking, and stepping. Interestingly, as soon as anyone practises BN, they appear to place the baby up their bodies even if there is no breastfeeding intent (like the father pictured below). Universal behaviour is a characteristic of an instinct, defined as an inborn or unlearned action, common to the species, having a fixed behavioural

Figure 40: Body Placing

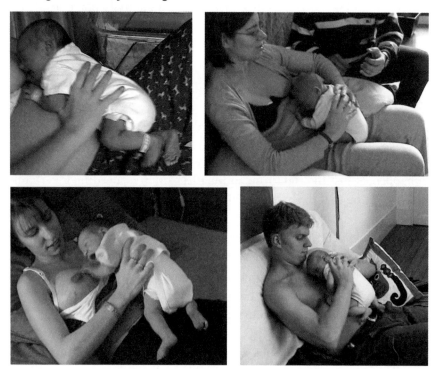

pattern without conscious intent.[5] The releaser of this behaviour appeared to be full-frontal contact independent of the state of dress.

Observe the intimate baby focus. As we've said previously, we know that even looking at a photo of a baby can release or increase oxytocin pulsatility. Gaze and imitation are well documented as spontaneous mother–baby behaviours in the human context, although they are not necessarily categorised as feeding behaviours. Looking again at video clip 6 below and, this time, focusing upon the mother's behaviours, you can see how she spontaneously opens her own mouth to show her baby how to latch.

Do you see that you cannot teach mothers to do this? Innate reproductive behaviours depend upon the right hormonal environment. That's where health professionals can play an important role. The BN approach emphasises the importance of maintaining an environment conducive to the release of the primary breastfeeding hormones: oxytocin and prolactin. No one else can protect mothers and babies the way midwives can.

Look at Video 8 to see how practising biological nurturing promotes mothers' self discovery. Supporting breastfeeding, using BN, enables health professionals to observe maternal behaviours, learning from mothers, and

Video 6: Mother spontaneously opens her mouth to show her baby how to latch

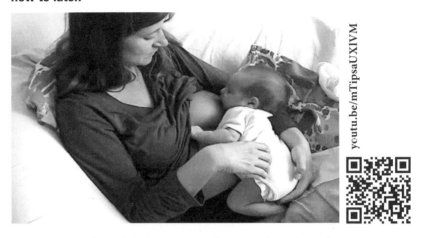

youtu.be/mTipsaUXIVM

You cannot teach mothers how to open their mouths and use their entire bodies to show their babies how to latch.

Video 8: Instinctive breastfeeding

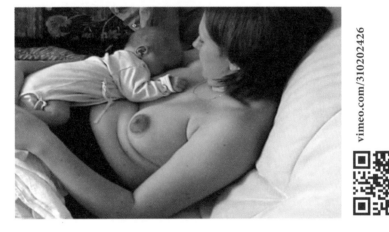

vimeo.com/310202426

I have not edited this clip, which reveals typical patterns of mother-baby pre-feed interactions. The mother has removed her blouse but this is not skin-to-skin contact as baby is lightly dressed. Mother and baby are complicit throughout absorbed in an intimate breastfeeding conversation.

trusting maternal instincts to release baby behaviours. That's exciting! There is no ceiling upon knowledge. There is so much more to learn. Today, despite some attempts to make breastfeeding a gender-neutral act, women are still the primary breastfeeders and providers of care for newborn babies, yet few women have ever been asked what they think. No mothers have ever been asked to participate in steering groups searching to define "instinct" in the human context.

In small groups, among BN Certified Breastfeeding Companions, we are currently working together to examine instinctual breastfeeding. There are some professional men in our groups, for example, medical doctors and pharmacists, but for the most part we are women, mothers.

So far, we can reliably assess veiling, a spontaneous, protective post-latching maternal behaviour that appears to reassure the mother and to communicate to the baby, through movement, that all is well. We have also reliably agreed spontaneous transportation, nesting, grooming, and identification behaviours specific to *Homo sapiens*. Watch this space.

CHAPTER 17

Biological Nurturing: A Mother-Centred Approach

Biological nurturing is a proactive mother-centred breastfeeding approach. The brand newborn baby is virtually always ready to be breast nurtured. Healthy term babies come into the world well fed. In physiological birth, the placenta is born as a result of welcoming the baby. Likewise, in physiological breastfeeding the maternal milk supply is the result of breast nurturing, not the reason to put the baby to breast.

Mothers wait for nine months to see and hold their babies. The first 48 to 72 hours are prime time. We do not need to be in a hurry. For countless numbers of mothers who have practised BN across the world, breastfeeding initiation was NOT responsive, not baby-led. Mothers didn't have to think or observe for cues. They didn't wait until the baby was awake nor did they apply gentle arousing strategies to awaken their babies to breastfeed.

Mothers didn't try to express their colostrum unless there was a reason. Instead, mothers were proactive, intuitively receiving tactile cues while nurturing their sleeping babies, cheek to breast – at the right address. Once mothers understand that during the first 48 to 72 hours their role is actually to take the lead, everything seems to come together.

Human mothers are amazing and very competent in their nurturing role. A proactive mothering style, however, is specific to the baby's age. Frequent, almost non-stop suckling during the first 48 to 72 hours is not only on the menu. It is the menu. It is virtually impossible to hold the baby too much. You can't spoil a baby or give her bad habits during that time. But it must be said that as the baby gets older, things evolve. Once breastfeeding is established, it's important to move towards a more responsive mothering style. As babies mature, they develop a capacity to self-soothe. At some point during the first six months, a mother will start to balance her own needs and her family's needs to conciliate them with the baby's.

However, during at least the first three days, the time of metabolic adaptation – a relatively short period – we want to encourage mothers to mimic womb feeding, keeping the sleeping baby at the right address. In doing so, mothers will recognise sooner when it's time to encourage self-soothing, differentiating when to be proactive or when to be responsive. In any case, parenting is always three steps forward and two steps back.

Importantly, the BN initial proactive approach aids metabolic adaptation by smoothing the inevitable discontinuity implicit in the transition from womb to world. There are untold benefits: babies who feed frequently during the first 24 hours maintain normal blood glucose levels. They often pass meconium sooner and experience less physiological jaundice later in the week.

Let us not forget that breastfeeding is more than milk. The very act of suckling reduces the risk of otitis media and broadens the baby's palatial arch. A proactive mothering style during the first three days helps mothers know their babies sooner. Close body nurturing often rescues any time lost through unexpected separation or difficulty and is associated with a copious milk supply.

There's a strong argument to suggest that one of the biggest threats to increasing breastfeeding rates is public health breastfeeding dogma that standardises mother–baby interactions, and midwifery policy enabling expressed breastmilk feeding during the first 48 to 72 hours. I conclude with some examples of these received ideas, contrasting them with the BN perspective.

Skin-to-skin contact is an especially lovely way to greet the baby, but it's not the only form of early mother–baby contact. It is quite possible that the protogaze – the first-time mothers establish eye-to-eye contact – is as important. Visual acuity is a mother's primary sense. Gazing and establishing comfortable eye-to-eye contact in as much naked contact as desired are immediate postpartum breastfeeding priorities.

On the postnatal ward, mothers should choose the form of early contact that best meets their needs and be encouraged to hold their sleeping babies as often as they desire.

Most health professionals assume that sleeping babies will not breastfeed. This received idea suggests that the sleeping baby is only safe when left in the plastic cot, separated from the "body learning." BN findings clearly indicate that this is not the case. Newborn babies latch on and feed with excellent milk transfer in sleep states.

Health professionals have been led to believe that hand expression is a useful tool. The UK BFI mandates teaching all mothers how to express their milk before hospital discharge. It has been widely assumed that hand expression stimulates mothers' milk production and increases breastfeeding duration. The research suggests otherwise. The biological nurturing perspective suggests that active suckling is important for both mother and baby, smoothing discontinuity from foetus to neonate, from pregnancy to postnatal.

Teaching all mothers to hand express keeps their babies at arm's length during prime suckling time. It also encourages passive feeding impeding the imprinting involved in the first breast latchments. This may distress babies and deregulate the mother's prolactin and oxytocin secretion often increasing maternal stress and anxiety. Stress and anxiety are breastfeeding enemies. The teaching of hand expression should be reserved for mothers of preterm babies and those who are separated from their babies.

Sitting bolt upright to breastfeed forces the newborn baby into a transverse lie, a malposition for most babies during foetal life. BN research demonstrates robust links between foetal and neonatal lie. Maintaining this continuity often promotes neonatal self-attachment. For any mother experiencing breastfeeding/latching difficulties, midwives should assess the neonate's lie in order to modify these positional indicators before suggesting hand expression.

Many midwives and lactation consultants suggest that an asymmetrical latch is the single most important variable associated with "correct" breast attachment enabling pain-free, effective breastfeeding. BN research clearly shows that the only correct latch is the one that is pain-free assuring good milk transfer. Just as there is not one correct position, there is not one correct latch. The BN latch is strongly associated with foetal attitude or the degree of flexion/extension in the womb. Before suggesting that mothers hand express, midwives should observe the baby's attitude during a breastfeed, aiming to ensure positional continuity from foetus to neonate.

Innate reproductive behaviours releasing instinctual behaviours depend upon an oxytocin environment. The role of midwives during the first 72 hours is to protect a mother's privacy, creating an environment conducive to the secretion of oxytocin and prolactin. Oxytocin is known as the "shy hormone," wary of teaching, showing, verbal instruction, questions, cold, bright lights, mundane conversation, fear, anxiety, pain, and discomfort. When mothers become repeatedly anxious, the worry and stress in itself may cause oxytocin to deregulate, creating a hormonal antithesis. Our maxim: "First, do no harm!"

Choice, continuity, and control were the three Cs of childbirth during the 1990s. Today, postnatal care remains the "Cinderella" of midwifery care. In view of static and low statistics of breastfeeding continuance, biological nurturing research suggests that it is time to apply the three Cs to postnatal care.

GLOSSARY

Behaviours

Actions, things you can see or hear, and describe objectively and reliably. In BN, we can describe reflex movements, states, and positions. For example, eyes moving under closed lids is one of the behaviours that characterise light sleep. Crying is also a behaviour because it is something you can hear. Descriptions like lazy, rude, or fussy are labels, not behaviours.

Biological nurturing

A form of early mother-baby contact promoting instinctual, mother-led breastfeeding. BN is more than a laid-back position. Mothers sit comfortably with their backs supported against the chair or sofa. The baby lies on top, sleeping cheek-to-breast or actively suckling. The degree of maternal recline optimises baby gazing and eye-to-eye contact. The baby's movements release some 20 primitive neonatal reflexes, aiding latch and milk transfer. Gazing and eye-to-eye contact release spontaneous maternal breastfeeding behaviours. Mother and baby actively participate.

BN

Abbreviation for biological nurturing. Like BF for breastfeeding, BN can be used as a noun or a verb. Examples: BN is a new breastfeeding approach. You can BN your baby when you're at home or out and about. BNing your baby often makes BF easier.

Biological nurturing continuum

Pregnancy, gestation, and birth are stages of reproductive life with a clear beginning and ending characterised by rupture, change, and separation. BN highlights golden nuggets of continuity hidden within five of its six components, smoothing neonatal adaptation and easing women into motherhood. *See continuity.*

Breast crawl

A form of skin-to-skin contact often encouraged in the immediate postpartum. Mothers, naked from the waist up, are placed lying flat on their backs. The naked or nappy-clad baby is placed in between her breasts with eyes at nipple level. A blanket often covers the baby's back. Mothers are asked not to shift the baby's position, but they are allowed to stroke and talk to their babies.

Continuity

The theoretical heart of biological nurturing. Foetal growth and development prepare neonatal behaviours aiding the transition from womb to world. For example, constant womb feeding prepares breastfeeding frequency during the first three days. Foetal lie in the womb prepares the way the baby spontaneously approaches the breast. Reflexes developed in the womb prepare the movements the baby uses to find the breast, latch, and suck. The dominant indeterminate sleep state in the womb is the optimal state for the baby to initiate breastfeeding.

Critical period

A developmental stage with a distinct beginning and ending. Experts suggest that the baby or child normally accomplishes at least one task before progressing to the next stage. Many believe that the first postnatal hour is a critical period; it is argued that there's increased and favoured sensitivity to maternal-infant bonding and establishing breastfeeding, and therefore, it is crucial for mothers and babies to be together during this time. BN highlights the sensitivity of the first 72 hours to accomplish these two tasks and extends this period to at least the first six weeks. *See Discontinuity.*

Description

In BN research, a systematic, objective account of mother-baby breastfeeding behaviours, positions, and maternal hormonal and neonatal behavioural states.

Discontinuity

Theory suggesting that children grow and develop during distinctly different stages. Similar to metamorphosis for some insects or amphibians, each stage has a change in habitat and behaviour, and is separate from the previous one. Once completed, you move on and you don't look back. *See critical period.*

Dorsal feeding positions

Traditional ways to hold babies based upon the widespread assumption that the human baby is an obligate dorsal feeder, whereby pressure is always required on the baby's back, neck, or head to keep him close to the breast. To counter gravitational effects, dorsal feeding positions are necessary when mothers lie on their sides or sit upright using the traditional baby holds: cradle, cross cradle, and rugby. In contrast, the BN research suggests that the human baby is a ventral feeder, like some of his mammalian cousins. *See frontal feeding positions.*

En face gazing

A form of intimate mother-baby contact where the mother places her baby's face just inches from her own face so that their eyes are in parallel alignment, optimising baby-gazing and eye-to-eye contact.

Frontal feeding positions

These are BN baby positions. The baby lies on top, tummy to mummy, with her entire torso, thighs, calves, and feet tops facing, touching, and closely applied either to her mother's body or to part of the environment as opposed to the traditional baby positions. *See dorsal feeding positions.*

Gestation

Always refers to the baby, meaning the baby's development from conception to birth in the womb. Lasts nine lunar months. Expected date of birth is normally assessed by ultrasound, which is not always accurate. Poor feeding is often linked to prematurity, and in BN positions, you can verify gestational age at a glance by observing the presence/absence and strength/amplitude of primitive neonatal reflexes, as well as the newborn baby's tone and attitude, or degree of flexion. Term babies are normally flexed, not hyperextended. *See neonatal attitude and primitive neonatal reflexes.*

Good Fit

A compact mother-baby, body-to-body apposition in the habitat of a behaving body. In BN, the baby lies prone but tilted upwards on a gentle maternal body slope. Good fit describes how well the baby's face and BN position is synchronised with his mother's breast and body. *See habitat.*

Gravity

The force attracting a body towards the centre of the earth. In BN, when mothers lay their babies on their bodies, gravitational pull helps to keep the baby close, whereas upright breastfeeding positions drag the baby down toward the pillow, toward the mum's lap or the floor. That is why mothers in vertical positions must apply pressure to baby's back to keep the baby closely applied to the breast. *See dorsal feeding positions.*

Habitat

A location or address, in space and in time of a life support system providing ambient temperature, humidity, light, and energy for growth and development of the offspring. In BN, the maternal habitat is the mother's mammary equipment and protective body. *See right breastfeeding address.*

Hawthorne Effect

This is a research bias that can distort findings. The Hawthorne effect occurs when the behaviour of research participants does not really represent what they usually do. Rather, participants try to please the researchers in whatever has been hypothesised. This is an unconscious reaction due to the fact that the participants know at the outset that they will be observed.

Hormonal complexion

Maternal features that regularly occur together that appear to characterise hormonal levels and pulsatility. We can recognise adrenalin, cortisol, and oxytocin because these emotional responses are often written all over people's facial expressions. Many women use make-up to create an oxytocin complexion enhancing sexual appeal. In BN, the role of the midwife is to create an environment where oxytocin, a shy hormone, dominates.

Instinctual breastfeeding

See biological nurturing.

Innate behaviours

Involuntary, inborn, instinctual, spontaneous actions or reactions. Things you can hear and see. Traditionally, experts have suggested that, at birth, the baby is hardwired to breastfeed, whereas mothers need to be taught breastfeeding skills and techniques because they lack innate behaviours. That claim doesn't make evolutionary sense. It is well-known that teaching suppresses instinctual response. In BN, the role of the midwife is to protect an environment conducive to high oxytocin pulsatility. An oxytocin environment underpins the release of innate behaviours.

Indeterminate sleep states

Dominate foetal and early neonatal life. Rapid transitions mean that behavioural state is not clearly defined. In BN positions, indeterminate sleep is an ideal state to initiate breastfeeding

Interpretation

An explanation or theory for a behaviour or phenomenon. Behaviour is open to many different interpretations and one researcher's clarifications can often enrich another's. Although based upon systematic, objective research observations, interpretation is always selective and personal to the researcher's experience. This means that the consumer of research (that's all of us) needs to be cautious not to consider any one researcher's behavioural interpretations as "the truth" (and that includes mine).

Latchment

Oral tactile imprinting occurring during the first stage of neonatal development. Term first coined by Australian Midwife Elsie Mobbs. Comprises early seeking behaviours of a sucking stimulus by the baby (for example, seeking the feel of the maternal nipple in the mouth). Once imprinted, the baby will experience emotional distress on the loss of such stimulus.

Laid-back breastfeeding

This is the biological nurturing maternal position. Breastfeeding in a semi-recumbent position uses gravity to aid latch and milk transfer. Mothers neither sit upright, nor do they lie flat on their backs. There is always a degree of recline, which ensures that the baby lies on top in a physiological body tilt. Neonatal positions, lying flat and prone, are associated with cot death, whereas the baby's BN tilted position enhances neonatal respiration

Maternal biological nurturing positions

See laid-back breastfeeding

Mechanisms (biological nurturing)

A system of mutually adapted parts working together. A means by which a particular effect is produced. Laid-back sitting postures and neonatal close ventral/frontal positions are the primary components of the BN system. Those two parts are "mutually adapted and working together" to release instinctual breastfeeding behaviours for both mothers and babies, even when babies are apparently in sleep states. Pressure from constant ventral contact releases movement, rippling to and fro from navel to limbs. Friction from the baby's limbs brushing against the mum, together with gravity, keeping the baby on top, are the means by which the particular effect or instinctual breastfeeding is produced.

Metabolic adaptation

Well orchestrated metabolic and hormonal adaptive changes that ensure a continuing supply of energy fuels. Ward-Platt and Deshpande define the science that should underpin early breastfeeding practice. As soon as the umbilical cord is cut, the continuous transplacental supply of glucose abruptly stops, the newborn must switch on the endogenous production of glucose until exogenous nutritional intake becomes established. The neonate then has to adjust to alternating periods of feeding and fasting. Metabolic adaptation lasts approximately three days. During the first 72 hours, frequent long episodes of BN maintain blood glucose concentrations within normal ranges. *See neonatal hypoglycaemia.*

Morphology

A particular form, shape, or body structure; the study of body shape and structure. In BN, maternal short-waisted morphology may be associated with the semi-reclined positions mothers use to optimise baby gazing and eye-to-eye contact while suckling their offspring.

Nature/Nurture Debate

Those supporting the nature perspective of the origins of behaviour argue that a person's capacity to act is inborn, not learned, rather a part of our genetic inheritance, built into the brain before birth. Advocates of the nurture determinant of behaviour consider that the baby is born like a clean slate ready for experiences and environmental learnings to write his behavioural capacity. Epidemiological variables, such as ethnicity, age, geographic situation, education, income, and social class are nurture. BN brings nature to the fore, attempting to restore balance, suggesting that under some biological circumstances, the capacity to breastfeed is innate, a part of our genetic inheritance. *See public health.*

Natural

A behaviour, skill, or quality that comes instinctively. Semi-reclined or laid-back maternal postures are not "natural" for human mothers. Rather, we are bipedal, and have a "natural" drive to be vertical. However, the human neonate is born a quadruped. The biological nurturing positions conciliate these opposing needs.

Navel radiation

Dominant pattern of baby movements in the womb, where movement ripples out from the centre, the navel, to head, sacrum or tail, and arms and legs in patterns similar to the radial symmetry found in the starfish. Movement remains organised around the navel for approximately the first 2 postnatal months.

Neonate

A newborn baby during the first month of life.

Neonatal attitude

Terminology borrowed from midwifery assessment of foetal attitude. The degree of flexion and/or extension ranging from the head and body, fully flexed (commonly called the foetal position) to the head or legs partially or fully extended. Babies in BN positions usually latch-on spontaneously when their position at the breast accommodates their foetal attitude. Assessment of neonatal attitude is also a way to confirm gestational age. *See gestational age.*

Neonatal biological nurturing positions

See full frontal feeding

Neonatal behavioural state

A group of behaviours that regularly occur together, indicating a level of arousal or neonatal consciousness. Although experts have identified up to nine states, the BN research used Brazelton's six states. However, in BN, drowsy is defined as a sleep state and I prefer the term "agitated" to describe the "fussy" state.

Neonatal lie

Terminology borrowed from midwifery assessment of foetal lie or the direction of the position. After birth, when mothers sit upright to breastfeed, the baby must lie in a transverse direction across her body. The transverse lie characterises a malposition during foetal life. If the lie remains transverse during labour, the mother will require a caesarean section. In BN, most babies attach spontaneously in either a longitudinal or oblique lie, the two normal positional directions during foetal life.

Nurture

Nurture means nourish, develop, raise, discipline, or educate. Nurturing behaviours are learned or acquired through imitation or environmental influences ranging from early feeding choices to opening a bank account for your child. Simply put, nurture is the culturally accepted way parents show their love for their babies. *See nature/nurture debate.*

Observations (biological nurturing)

Data collection method. Researchers receive knowledge through the senses (vision and auditory senses dominate. BN videotaped observations were systematic. That is, they commenced as soon as mothers picked their babies up with feeding intention. After five minutes, if the baby had not attached, positional changes were suggested. Videotapes were viewed and reviewed, where reflexes, positions, and behavioural states were described objectively among a group of five experts. *See validity and reliability.*

Plasticity

Describes the human capacity for change in response to a positive or negative environment where life experiences can mould growth and development. The environment can enrich or impoverish the human capacity to establish crucial competencies and achieve developmental milestones. Previously thought to be limited to critical periods, plasticity is now known to occur over time. Practising BN during the first three days is the right environment to enhance breastfeeding and bonding.

Pregnancy

Being with child, carrying the developing embryo or foetus in the womb. Always applies to the mother. During pregnancy, mothers have a tactile communication with their babies. For example, the baby kicks, the mum responds. From a BN perspective, once born, mothers know more about their babies than anyone else. Mothers are amazing and we midwives need to observe and learn from them.

Primitive neonatal reflexes

Inborn, unconditioned, involuntary reactions or responses to endogenous or environmental stimuli. Develop in utero from 28 gestational weeks. Paediatricians evaluate reflexes as a screening test for neurological function and to predict gestational age. During BN, sustained close ventral contact with the mother's body curves releases navel radiation. Body brushing and spontaneous maternal releasing behaviours (like playing with the baby's feet) release some 20 reflexes, appearing to have breastfeeding function. *See navel radiation and the mechanisms of BN.*

Protogaze

Translated from "protoregard," an expression coined by Marc Pilliot, French paediatrician. From the Greek "protos," meaning first in time or place. Biological nurturing positions optimise the first gaze and the first-time mothers and babies establish eye-to-eye contact. Both are powerful releasers of innate behaviours.

Public Health

The science of health promotion, informed by epidemiology. Education, consistency in policies, and legislation nudges consumers toward healthy choices and lifestyles, and protects the public from disease and injury. Seatbelts are a prime example, standardising instructions, saving millions of lives each year. Breastfeeding is an important public health issue, reducing short and long-term infant and maternal morbidity. Epidemiological studies suggest targeting disadvantaged groups based on personal and socioeconomic factors. BN supports the need for a strong public health breastfeeding approach to promote, educate, and legislate but suggests that, unlike the compulsory wearing of seatbelts, breastfeeding initiation cannot be standardised into a one-size-fits-all approach.

Reliability (Research and Practice)

The degree to which health professionals making the same assessment at the same time consistently obtain the same result. For example, two sales persons using a yardstick that measures 35 inches to sell a yard of material will reliably measure the cloth. However, the customer who needs a yard will be shortchanged because the rod does not measure what it purports to measure. Likewise, breastfeeding tools often include latch assessment. When two or more practitioners assess the same baby at the same time, they can reliably identify the "correct" latch. However, that does not mean that the "correct" latch is a valid measure of milk transfer. *See validity.*

Right breastfeeding address

The developmental habitat, including the mother's womb, her body, and her lactational apparatus, optimising learning from a behaving body. BN argues that learning via a behaving body is mutual and has nothing to do with dress state. Close body contact with her baby not only releases inborn baby behaviours but also develops the mother's capacity to breastfeed instinctually. For this to happen, the human baby is not lying under the mum's chin, neither low on her abdomen, nor between her breasts. The human baby is either suckling actively on the breast or sleeping cheek-to-breast. *See habitat.*

Sign stimulus

A colour, position, or behaviour releasing an innate act. The BN argument suggests that baby gazing and eye-to-eye contact are powerful sign stimuli releasing innate maternal breastfeeding behaviours or instinctual breastfeeding.

Skin-to-skin contact

A form of early mother-baby contact, where the mother is naked from the waist up and holds her naked or nappy-clad baby in close ventral contact. *See the breast crawl.*

Sucking

Used as an adjective means not weaned or very young. As a verb, sucking is an inborn neonatal feeding reflex. Although the primary function is milk transfer, babies have a strong sucking drive and both nutritive and non-nutritive sucking satisfies this. Although the need is best satisfied through early breast latchment and nutritive and non-nutritive breast suckling. *See latchment.*

Suckling

Breast nurturing, something that both mothers and babies do. Mothers' suckling behaviours release foot reflexes. Mothers also spontaneously form their nipples, and/ or compress their breasts. When they place their sleeping babies cheek to breast, they often make an airway and/or coordinate the latch without guidance. They smile, laugh, groom, imitate, and talk to their babies. Mothers' spontaneous suckling behaviours are amazing. Babies' suckling behaviours include sleeping, licking, mouthing, rooting, pushing-up, sucking in bursts (nutritive sucking), and occasional sucking or flutter feeding (non-nutritive sucking). Babies' spontaneous suckling behaviours are amazing.

Validity (Research and Practice)

A research instrument or tool, like a breastfeeding assessment, measures what it says it measures. A yardstick that is 35 inches long may look like a yardstick, but it does not measure a yard. The BN perspective suggests that the correct (asymmetric) latch does not measure milk transfer. An invalid tool can be reliable. *See Reliability.*

Womb feeding

During gestation, the constant transfer of glucose and nutrients via the umbilical cord. As soon as the cord is cut at birth, this stops. The baby must now adapt to a feeding fasting pattern. The BN argument suggests that during this transition, mothers can keep their sleeping babies cheek to breast to increase early small frequent breastfeeds. *See metabolic adaptation.*

REFERENCES

CHAPTER 1: WHAT IS BIOLOGICAL NURTURING?

1. Colson, S. (2008). Bringing nature to the fore. *Practising Midwife, 11*(10), 14-16, 18-19.
2. Sulcova, E. (1997). *Prague Newborn Behaviour Description Technique: Manual.* Prague: Psychiatric Centre, Laboratory of Psychometric Studies.
3. Colson, S. (2006). *The mechanisms of biological nurturing.* PhD dissertation, Canterbury Christ Church University, Canterbury, UK.
4. Page, D. (2007). Breastfeeding: Learning the dance of latching. *Journal of Human Lactation, 23*(1), 111-112.
5. Smillie, C., Frantz, K., & Makelin, I. (2005). *Baby-led breastfeeding the mother-baby dance* [DVD]. Retrieved from http://www.geddesproduction.com/breast-feeding-baby-lcd.php
6. Alberts, J.R. (1994). Learning as adaptation of the infant. *Acta Paediatrica,* 397(supplement), 77–85.
7. Pollard, M. (2017). *Evidence-based care for breastfeeding mothers.* Abingdon, UK: Routledge.

CHAPTER 2: WHY DO WE NEED A NEW BREASTFEEDING APPROACH?

1. Burns E., Fenwick, J., Sheehan, A., & Schmied, V. (2013). Mining for liquid gold: Midwifery language and practices associated with early breastfeeding support. *Maternal and Child Nutrition, 9,* 57–73.
2. Righard, L., & Alade, M.O. (1990). Effects of delivery room routines on success of first feed. *The Lancet, 336,* 1105-1107.
3. Morris, D. (1977). *Manwatching: A field guide to human behaviour.* London: Triad/Panther Ltd.
4. Lorenz, K. (1952). *King Solomon's ring.* London: Methuen & Co Ltd.
5. Tinbergen, N. (1951). *The study of instinct.* Oxford: Clarendon Press.
6. Slater, A., & Bremner, J.G. (2017). *An introduction to developmental psychology,* 3rd Ed. Chichester, UK: John Wiley & Sons Ltd.
7. Baggott, R. (2011). *Public health policy and politics,* 2nd Ed. London: Palgrave Macmillan.
8. Cadogan, W. (1748). *An essay upon nursing, and the management of children: From their birth to three years of age.* London: Published by Order of the General Committee for transacting the Affairs of the Foundling Hopsital. Reprinted for J. Roberts in Warwick-Lane. p.3
9. Hardyment, C. (1983). *Dream babies: Child care from Locke to Spock.* London: Jonathan Cape.
10. Truby King, F.T. (1924). *The expectant mother, and baby's first months.* London: Macmillan. p. 55
11. Truby King, M. (1934) *Mothercraft.* London: Simpkin, Marshall Ltd., p. 4
12. Slater, A., & Bremner, J.G. (2017). *An introduction to developmental psychology,* 3rd Ed. Chichester, UK: John Wiley & Sons Ltd.
13. Gunther, M. (1955). Instinct and the nursing couple. *Lancet, 265,* 575-578.
14. Pryor, K. (1963). *Nursing your baby* (1st Ed.). New York: Harper & Row., p. 69)
15. Inch, S. (2014). Infant feeding. In J.E. Marshall & M.D. Raynor (Eds.), *Myles textbook for midwives,* 16th Ed. London: Churchill Livingstone Elsevier.
16. Burns E., Fenwick, J., Sheehan, A., & Schmied, V. (2013). Mining for liquid gold: Midwifery language and practices associated with early breastfeeding support. *Maternal and Child Nutrition, 9,* 57–73. p. 62
17. Entwistle, F. (2013). *The evidence and rationale for the UNICEF UK Baby Friendly Initiative standards* (p. 74). London: UNICEF UK.
18. Inch, S. (2014). Infant feeding. In J.E. Marshall & M.D. Raynor (Eds.), *Myles textbook for midwives,* 16th Ed. London: Churchill Livingstone Elsevier.
19. UNICEF UK. (2010). *The Baby-Friendly Initiative.* Retrieved from http://www.babyfriendly.org.uk.
20. Moore, E.R., Bergman, N., Anderson, G.C., & Medley, N. (2016). *Early skin-to-skin contact*

for mothers and their healthy newborn infants. Cochrane Database of Systematic Reviews, 11. Retrieved from www.cochranelibrary.com

21. Entwistle, F. (2013). *The evidence and rationale for the UNICEF UK Baby Friendly Initiative standards* (p. 74). London: UNICEF UK.
22. Inch, S. (2014). Infant feeding. In J.E. Marshall & M.D. Raynor (Eds.), *Myles textbook for midwives*, 16th Ed. London: Churchill Livingstone Elsevier.
23. Colson, S. (2008). Bringing nature to the fore. *Practising Midwife, 11*(10), 14-16, 18-19.

CHAPTER 3: THE ROOTS OF BIOLOGICAL NURTURING

1. Colson, S. (1997). A baby feeding advisor: Who needs one? *Midwifery Matters, 72*, 14-17.
2. Hartmann, P.E., & Prosser, C.G. (1984). Physiological basis of longitudinal changes in human milk yield and composition. *Federation Proceedings, 43*, 2448-2453.
3. Hartmann, P.E. (1987). Lactation and reproduction in Western Australian women. *Reproductive Medicine, 32*, 543-547.
4. De Rooy, L., & Hawdon, J.M. (2002). Nutritional factors that affect the postnatal metabolic adaptation of full-term small and large for gestational age infants. *Pediatrics, 109*, 42. Retrieved from http://pediatrics.aappublications.org/cgi/content/full/109/3/e42.
5. Hawdon, J.M., Ward-Platt, M.P., & Aynsley-Green, A. (1992). Patterns of metabolic adaptation in term and preterm infants in the first postnatal week. *Archives of Diseases of Childhood, 67*, 357-365.
6. Righard, L., & Frantz, K. (1992). *Delivery self attachment* [video]. Sunland, CA: Geddes Productions.
7. Bragg, M. (1991). Review and abstract. Righard L. & Alade, M.O. (1990). Effect of delivery room routines on success of first breast-feed. *Lancet, 336*, 8723, 1105-1107in MIDIRS Midwifery Digest Review No. 901031 Standard Search L46, PN101. Retrieved from http://www.MIDIRS.org
8. World Health Organization (WHO). (1998). *Evidence for the ten steps to successful breastfeeding* (Revised). Family and Reproductive Health Division of Child Health and Development. Geneva: World Health Organization.
9. Ludington-Hoe, S.M., with Golant, S.K. (1993). *Kangaroo care.* New York: Bantam Books.
10. De Rooy, L., & Hawdon, J.M. (2002). Nutritional factors that affect the postnatal metabolic adaptation of full-term small and large for gestational age infants. *Pediatrics, 109*, 42. Retrieved from http://pediatrics.aappublications.org/cgi/content/full/109/3/e42.
11. Hawdon, J.M., Ward-Platt, M.P., & Aynsley-Green, A. (1992). Patterns of metabolic adaptation in term and preterm infants in the first postnatal week. *Archives of Diseases of Childhood, 67*, 357-365.
12. Hoseth, E., Joergensen, A., Ebbesen, F., & Moeller, M. (2000). Blood glucose levels in a population of healthy breastfed term infants of appropriate size for gestational age. *Archives of Diseases of Childhood: Foetal Neonatal Edition, 83*, F117-F119.
13. Colson, S., & Giffiths, H. (1996). Breastfeeding: Rediscovery of the lost art. *Nursing Times, 92*(11), 59-64.
14. Colson, S. (1997). A baby feeding advisor: Who needs one? *Midwifery Matters, 72*, 14-17.

CHAPTER 4: THE BIOLOGICAL NURTURING CONTINUUM

1. Slater, A., & Bremner, J.G. (2017). *An introduction to developmental psychology*, 3rd Ed. Chichester, UK: John Wiley & Sons Ltd.
2. Baston, H. (2014). Antenatal care. In J.E. Marshall & M.D. Raynor (Eds.), *Myles textbook for midwives*, 16th Ed. London: Churchill Livingstone Elsevier.
3. Colson, S. (2006). *The mechanisms of biological nurturing.* PhD dissertation, Canterbury Christ Church University, Canterbury, UK.
4. Colson, S.D. (2014). Does the mother's posture have a protective role to play during skin-to-skin contact? Research observations and theories? *Clinical Lactation, 5*(2), 41-50.
5. Fleming P.J., Blair, P.S., Bacon, C., Bensley, D., Smith, I., Taylor, E., & Tripp, J. (1996). Environment of infants during sleep and risk of the sudden infant death syndrome: Results of 1993-1995 case-control study for confidential inquiry into stillbirths and deaths

in infancy. Confidential enquiry into stillbirths and deaths regional coordinators and researchers. *British Medical Journal, 313*, 191–195.

6. Skadberg, B. T., Morild, I., & Markestad, T. (1998). Abandoning prone sleeping: Effects on the risk of sudden infant death syndrome. *Journal of Pediatrics, 132*, 340–343.

7. Bainbridge, C.B. (1986). *The evolutionary origins of movement*. Amherst MA: School for Body-Mind Centring.

8. Masgutova, S., with Akhmatova, N. (2004). *Integration of dynamic and postural reflexes into the whole-body movement system*. Warsaw: International Neurokinesiology Institute. Retrieved from http://www.masgutovamethod.com.

9. Nowak, K., & Sendrowski, K. (2016). Neurophysiological aspects of neurotactile therapy of Masgutova Neurosensory Motor Reflex Integration. *Medical Rehabilitation, 20*(4), 1-10. Retrieved from http://www.masgutovamethod.com.

10. Landon, P., & Cazals, B. (2016). *La kinésphère réflexes de vue et réflexes faciaux*. Caen, France: Le Plaisir d'Apprendre.

11. Bainbridge, C.B. (1986). *The evolutionary origins of movement*. Amherst MA: School for Body-Mind Centring.

12. Mirmiran, M., Maas, Y.G.H., & Ariagno, R.L. (2003). Development of foetal and neonatal sleep and circadian rhythms. *Sleep Medicine Reviews, 7*(4), 321-334.

13. Einspieler, C., & Prechtl, H.F.R. (2005). Prechtl's Assessment of General Movements: A diagnostic tool for the functional assessment of the young nervous system. *Mental Retardation and Developmental Disabilities Research Reviews, 11, 61–67.*

14. Goddard-Blythe, S. (2008). *What babies and children really need*. Gloucestershire, UK: Hawthorn Press.

15. Brazelton, T.B., & Nugent, K. (2011). *Neonatal Behavioural Assessment Scale* (4th Ed.). London: MacKeith Press.

16. Inch, S. (2014). Infant feeding. In J.E. Marshall & M.D. Raynor (Eds.), *Myles textbook for midwives*, 16th Ed. London: Churchill Livingstone Elsevier.

17. Colson, S., DeRooy, L., & Hawdon, J. (2003). Biological nurturing increases breastfeeding duration. *MIDIRS Midwifery Digest, 13*(1), 92-97.

18. Einspieler, C., & Prechtl, H.F.R. (2005). Prechtl's Assessment of General Movements: A diagnostic tool for the functional assessment of the young nervous system. *Mental Retardation and Developmental Disabilities Research Reviews, 11, 61–67.*

19. Brazelton, T.B., & Nugent, K. (2011). *Neonatal Behavioural Assessment Scale* (4th Ed.). London: MacKeith Press.

20. Peiper, A. (1963). *Cerebral function in infancy and childhood* (3rd Ed.) B. Nagler & H. Nagler (Trans.). New York: Consultants Bureau.

21. Nijhuis, J.G., Prechtl, H.F., Martin, C.B., Jr., & Bots, R.S. (1982). Are there behavioural states in the human foetus? *Early Human Development, 6*, 177-195.

22. Brazelton T.B. (1961). Psychophysiologic reactions in the neonate. 1: The value of observation of the neonate. *Journal of Pediatrics, 58*, 508-512.

23. Brazelton, T.B., & Nugent, K. (2011). *Neonatal Behavioural Assessment Scale* (4th Ed.). London: MacKeith Press.

24. Mirmiran, M., Maas, Y.G.H., & Ariagno, R.L. (2003). Development of foetal and neonatal sleep and circadian rhythms. *Sleep Medicine Reviews, 7*(4), 321-334.

25. Biancuzzo, M. (1999). *Breastfeeding the newborn. Clinical strategies for nurses*. St Louis, MO: Mosby.

26. Blackburn, S.T. (2012). *Maternal, foetal, and neonatal physiology: A clinical perspective* (2nd Ed.). St Louis, MO: W.B. Saunders Company.

27. Entwistle, F. (2013). *The evidence and rationale for the UNICEF UK Baby Friendly Initiative standards* (p. 74). London: UNICEF UK.

28. Riordan, J., & Hoover, K. (2010). Perinatal and intrapartum care. In J. Riordan & K. Wambach (Eds.), *Breastfeeding and human lactation* (4th Ed.). Boston, MA: Jones & Bartlett.

29. Gadroy, D. (2016). *Naturellement votre. Mémoire de diplôme universitaire en lactation humaine et allaitement materne* (DIULHAM). Retrieved

from http://www.societe-francaise-neonatalogie.fr/2016/07/04/
diu-lactation-humaine-allaitement-maternel-diulham/

30. De Gasquet, B. (2005). *Bébé est la, vive maman, les suites de couches*. Paris: Robert Jauze.
31. McNabb, M., & Colson, S. (2000). From pregnancy to lactation: Changing relations between mother and baby/a biological perspective. In J. Alexander, C. Roth, & V. Levy (Eds.). *Midwifery Practice Core Topics, 3*, 51-65.
32. Uvnäs Moberg, K. (2003). *The oxytocin factor*. Cambridge, MA: Da Capo Press.
33. Nissen, E., Uvnäs Moberg, K., Svensson, K., Stock, S., Widstrom, A.M., & Winberg, J. (1996). Different patterns of oxytocin, prolactin but not cortisol release during breastfeeding in women delivered by Caesarean section or by the vaginal route. *Early Human Development, 45*, 103-118.
34. Bullough, C.H.W., Msuku, R.S., & Karonde, L. (1989). Early suckling and postpartum haemorrhage: Controlled trial in deliveries by traditional birth attendants. *The Lancet, 9*, 522-525.
35. Nissen, E., Uvnäs Moberg, K., Svensson, K., Stock, S., Widstrom, A.M., & Winberg, J. (1996). Different patterns of oxytocin, prolactin but not cortisol release during breastfeeding in women delivered by Caesarean section or by the vaginal route. *Early Human Development, 45*, 103-118.
36. Alberts, J.R., & Cramer C.P. (1988). Ecology and experience. In E.M. Blass (Ed.), *Developmental psychobiology and behavioural ecology. Handbook of behavioural neurobiology, Vol 9*. Boston, MA: Springer.

CHAPTER 5: KEEP THE BABY AT THE RIGHT ADDRESS

1. Alberts, J.R. (1994). Learning as adaptation of the infant. *Acta Paediatrica, 397*(supplement), 77–85.
2. Alberts, J.R., & Cramer C.P. (1988). Ecology and experience. In E.M. Blass (Ed.), *Developmental psychobiology and behavioural ecology. Handbook of behavioural neurobiology, Vol 9*. Boston, MA: Springer.
3. Alberts, J.R. (1994). Learning as adaptation of the infant. *Acta Paediatrica, 397*(supplement), 77–85.
4. ibid
5. ibid
6. Colson, S. (2002). Womb to world: A metabolic perspective. *Midwifery Today, 46*(1), 12-17.
7. De Rooy, L., & Hawdon, J.M. (2002). Nutritional factors that affect the postnatal metabolic adaptation of full-term small and large for gestational age infants. *Pediatrics, 109*, 42. Retrieved from http://pediatrics.aappublications.org/cgi/content/full/109/3/e42.
8. Hawdon, J.M., Ward-Platt, M.P., & Aynsley-Green, A. (1992). Patterns of metabolic adaptation in term and preterm infants in the first postnatal week. *Archives of Diseases of Childhood, 67*, 357-365.
9. De Rooy, L., & Hawdon, J.M. (2002). Nutritional factors that affect the postnatal metabolic adaptation of full-term small and large for gestational age infants. *Pediatrics, 109*, 42. Retrieved from http://pediatrics.aappublications.org/cgi/content/full/109/3/e42.
10. Hawdon, J.M., Ward-Platt, M.P., & Aynsley-Green, A. (1992). Patterns of metabolic adaptation in term and preterm infants in the first postnatal week. *Archives of Diseases of Childhood, 67*, 357-365.
11. Hoseth, E., Joergensen, A., Ebbesen, F., & Moeller, M. (2000). Blood glucose levels in a population of healthy breastfed term infants of appropriate size for gestational age. *Archives of Diseases of Childhood: Foetal Neonatal Edition, 83*, F117-F119.
12. Colson, S. (2000). *Biological suckling facilitates exclusive breastfeeding from birth a pilot study of twelve vulnerable infants*. Unpublished master's dissertation. London: South Bank University.
13. Colson, S., DeRooy, L., & Hawdon, J. (2003). Biological nurturing increases breastfeeding duration. *MIDIRS Midwifery Digest, 13*(1), 92-97.
14. ibid
15. Moore, E.R., Bergman, N., Anderson, G.C., & Medley, N. (2016). *Early skin-to-skin contact*

for mothers and their healthy newborn infants. Cochrane Database of Systematic Reviews, 11. Retrieved from www.cochranelibrary.com

16. Widström, A. M., Lilja, G., Aaltomaa-Michalias, P., Dahllof, A., Lintula, M., & Nissen, E. (2011). Newborn behaviour to locate the breast when skin-to-skin: A possible method for enabling early self-regulation. *Acta Paediatrica Scandinavica, 100,* 79–85.

17. Righard, L. (2008) The baby is breastfeeding—not the mother. *Birth, 35*(1), 1-2.

18. Salk, L. (1973). The role of heartbeat in relations between mother and infant. *Scientific American, 228,* 24-29.

19. Morris, D. (1977). *Manwatching: A field guide to human behaviour.* London: Triad/Panther Ltd.

20. Righard, L., & Alade, M O. (1990). Effects of delivery room routines on success of first feed. *The Lancet, 336,* 1105-1107.

21. Widström, A. M., Lilja, G., Aaltomaa-Michalias, P., Dahllof, A., Lintula, M., & Nissen, E. (2011). Newborn behaviour to locate the breast when skin-to-skin: A possible method for enabling early self-regulation. *Acta Paediatrica Scandinavica, 100,* 79–85.

22. Bullough, C.H.W., Msuku, R.S., & Karonde, L. (1989). Early suckling and postpartum haemorrhage: Controlled trial in deliveries by traditional birth attendants. *The Lancet, 9,* 522-525.

23. Widström, A. M., Lilja, G., Aaltomaa-Michalias, P., Dahllof, A., Lintula, M., & Nissen, E. (2011). Newborn behaviour to locate the breast when skin-to-skin: A possible method for enabling early self-regulation. *Acta Paediatrica Scandinavica, 100,* 79–85.

24. Klaus, M.H., & Kennel, J.H. (1976). *Maternal-infant bonding* (1st American Ed.). St Louis, MO: Mosby Company.

CHAPTER 6: TRANSITIONS: COPING WITH DISCONTINUITY

1. Blackburn, S.T. (2012). *Maternal, foetal, and neonatal physiology: A clinical perspective* (2nd Ed.). St Louis, MO: W.B. Saunders Company.

2. Ward-Platt, M., & Deshpande, S. (2005). Metabolic adaptation at birth. *Seminars in Foetal & Neonatal Medicine, 10,* 341-350, p. 341

3. Hawdon, J.M. (2013). Definition of neonatal hypoglycaemia, time for a rethink? *Archives of Diseases of Childhood: Foetal Neonatal Ed., 98*(5), F382-F383.

4. Ward-Platt, M., & Deshpande, S. (2005). Metabolic adaptation at birth. *Seminars in Foetal & Neonatal Medicine, 10,* 341-350, p. 341

5. Cornblath, M., Hawdon, J.M., Williams, A.F., Aynsley-Green,A., Ward-Platt, M., Schwartz, R., & Kalhan, S.C. (2000). Controversies regarding definition of neonatal hypoglycaemia: Suggested operational thresholds. *Pediatrics, 105,* 1141–1145.

6. De Rooy, L., & Hawdon, J.M. (2002). Nutritional factors that affect the postnatal metabolic adaptation of full-term small and large for gestational age infants. *Pediatrics, 109,* 42. Retrieved from http://pediatrics.aappublications.org/cgi/content/full/109/3/e42.

7. Hawdon, J.M. (2012). Disorders of metabolic homeostasis in the neonate. In J.M. Rennie (Ed.), *Textbook of neonatology* (pp. 850-867). Edinburgh, UK: Churchill Livingstone, Elsevier.

8. Hawdon, J.M. (2013). Definition of neonatal hypoglycaemia, time for a rethink? *Archives of Diseases of Childhood: Fetal Neonatal Ed., 98*(5), F382-F383.

9. Hawdon, J.M. (1993). Diabetes and neonatal hypoglycaemia: The consequences of admission to the special care nursery. *Maternal Child Health,* 48–51.

10. Ward-Platt, M., & Deshpande, S. (2005). Metabolic adaptation at birth. *Seminars in Foetal & Neonatal Medicine, 10,* 341-350, p. 341

11. Alberts, J.R. (1994). Learning as adaptation of the infant. *Acta Paediatrica,* 397(supplement), 77–85.

12. Moore, E.R., Bergman, N., Anderson, G.C., & Medley, N. (2016). *Early skin-to-skin contact for mothers and their healthy newborn infants.* Cochrane Database of Systematic Reviews, 11. Retrieved from www.cochranelibrary.com

13. Holmes, A.V., McLeod, A.Y., & Bunik, M. (2013). ABM Clinical Protocol #5: Peripartum

breastfeeding management for the healthy mother and infant at term. *Breastfeeding Medicine*, 8(6), 469-473. Retrieved from https://www.bfmed.org/protocols.

14. Widström, A. M., Lilja, G., Aaltomaa-Michalias, P., Dahllof, A., Lintula, M., & Nissen, E. (2011). Newborn behaviour to locate the breast when skin-to-skin: A possible method for enabling early self-regulation. *Acta Paediatrica Scandinavica, 100*, 79–85.

15. Holmes, A.V., McLeod, A.Y., & Bunik, M. (2013). ABM Clinical Protocol #5: Peripartum breastfeeding management for the healthy mother and infant at term. *Breastfeeding Medicine*, 8(6), 469-473. Retrieved from https://www.bfmed.org/protocols.

16. The Public Health Agency. (2018). *Breastfeeding advice and guidance.* Retrieved from https://www.breastfedbabies.org/breastfeeding-advice-and-guidance.

17. UNICEF UK Baby Friendly Initiative. (2017). *Guide to the UNICEF-UK Baby-Friendly Initiative standards* (2nd Ed.). London: UNICEF.

18. Entwistle, F. (2013). *The evidence and rationale for the UNICEF UK Baby Friendly Initiative standards* (p. 74). London: UNICEF UK.

19. Morton, J. (2017). *Early hand expression increases later milk production.* Retrieved from https://med.stanford.edu/newborns/professional-education/breastfeeding/hand-expressing-milk.html.

20. UNICEF UK Baby Friendly Initiative. (2017). *Guide to the UNICEF-UK Baby-Friendly Initiative standards* (2nd Ed.). London: UNICEF.

21. Morton, J. (2017). *Early hand expression increases later milk production.* Retrieved from https://med.stanford.edu/newborns/professional-education/breastfeeding/hand-expressing-milk.html.

22. ibid

23. Flaherman, V.J., Gay, B., Scott, C., Avins, A., Lee, K.A., & Newman, T.B. (2012a). Randomised trial comparing hand expression with breast pumping for mothers of term newborns feeding poorly. *Archives of Diseases of Childhood: Foetal and Neonatal Ed., 97*(1), F18–F23.

24. Zinaman, M.J., Hughes, V., Queenan, J.T., Labbok, M.H., & Albertson, B. (1992). Acute prolactin and oxytocin responses and milk yield to infant suckling and artificial methods of expression in lactating women. *Pediatrics, 89*, 437–440.

25. UNICEF UK Baby Friendly Initiative. (2017). *Guide to the UNICEF-UK Baby-Friendly Initiative standards* (2nd Ed.). London: UNICEF.

26. Flaherman, V.J., Gay, B., Scott, C., Avins, A., Lee, K.A., & Newman, T.B. (2012a). Randomised trial comparing hand expression with breast pumping for mothers of term newborns feeding poorly. *Archives of Diseases of Childhood: Foetal and Neonatal Ed., 97*(1), F18–F23.

27. Entwistle, F. (2017). Infant feeding and relationship building. In S. MacDonald & G. Johnson (Eds.), *Mayes midwifery*, 15th Ed. (pp. 757-787). Edinburgh: Elsevier.

28. Forster, D.A., Johns, H.M., McLachlan, H.L., Moorhead, A.M., McEgan, K.M., & Amir, L.H. (2015). Feeding infants directly at the breast during the postpartum hospital stay is associated with increased breastfeeding at 6 months postpartum: A prospective cohort study. *BMJ, 5*, e007512. doi:10.1136/bmjopen-2014- 007512

29. Clemons, S.N., & Amir, L.H. (2010). Breastfeeding women's experience of 39. expressing: A descriptive study. *Journal of Human Lactation, 26*, 258–265.

30. Geraghty, S.R., Khoury, J.C., & Kalkwarf, H.J. (2005). Human milk pumping rates of mothers of singletons and mothers of multiples. *Journal of Human Lactation, 21*, 413–420.

31. Hornbeak, D.M., Dirani, M., Sham, W.K., Li, J., Young, T.L., Wong, T.Y., Chong, Y.S., & Saw, S.M. (2010). Emerging trends in breastfeeding practices in Singaporean Chinese women: Findings from a population-based study. *Annals of Academic Medicine, 39*, 88–94.

32. Labiner-Wolfe, J., Fein, S.B., Shealy, K.R., & Wang, C. (2008). Prevalence of breast milk expression and associated factors. *Pediatrics, 122*(Suppl 2), S63–S68.

33. Shealy, K.R., Scanlon, K.S., Labiner-Wolfe, J., Fein, S.B., & Grummer-Strawn, L.M. (2008). Characteristics of 38 breastfeeding practices among US mothers. *Pediatrics, 122*(Suppl 2), S50–S55.

34. Win, N.N., Binns, C., Zhao, Y., Scott, J.A., & Oddy, W.H. (2006). Breastfeeding duration

in mothers who express breast milk: A cohort study. *International Breastfeeding Journal,* *1*, 28.

35. Meehan, K., Harrison, G.G., Afifi, A.A., Nickel, N., Jenks, E., & Ramirez, A. (2008). The association between a 35 electric pump loan program and the timing of requests for formula by working mothers in WIC. *Journal of Human Lactation, 24*, 150–158.

36. Win, N.N., Binns, C., Zhao, Y., Scott, J.A., & Oddy, W.H. (2006). Breastfeeding duration in mothers who express breast milk: A cohort study. *International Breastfeeding Journal,* *1*, 28.

37. Geraghty, S.R., Khoury, J.C., & Kalkwarf, H.J. (2005). Human milk pumping rates of mothers of singletons and mothers of multiples. *Journal of Human Lactation, 21*, 413–420.

38. Schwartz, K., D'Arcy, H.J., Gillespie, B., Bobo, J., Longeway, M., & Foxman, B. (2002). Factors associated with weaning in the first 3 months postpartum. *Journal of Family Practice, 51*, 439–444.

39. Forster, D.A., Johns, H.M., McLachlan, H.L., Moorhead, A.M., McEgan, K.M., & Amir, L.H. (2015). Feeding infants directly at the breast during the postpartum hospital stay is associated with increased breastfeeding at 6 months postpartum: A prospective cohort study. *BMJ, 5*, e007512. doi:10.1136/bmjopen-2014- 007512

40. Zinaman, M.J., Hughes, V., Queenan, J.T., Labbok, M.H., & Albertson, B. (1992). Acute prolactin and oxytocin responses and milk yield to infant suckling and artificial methods of expression in lactating women. *Pediatrics, 89*, 437–440.

41. Lawrence, R.A., & Lawrence, R.M. (2011). *Breastfeeding: A guide for the medical profession,* 7th Ed. Maryland Heights, MI: Mosby.

42. Mobbs, E. (2011). *Latchment before attachment: The first stage of emotional development oral tactile imprinting.* Westmead, Australia: G.T. Crarf Pty Ltd.

43. Zinaman, M.J., Hughes, V., Queenan, J.T., Labbok, M.H., & Albertson, B. (1992). Acute prolactin and oxytocin responses and milk yield to infant suckling and artificial methods of expression in lactating women. *Pediatrics, 89*, 437–440.

44. Holmes, A.V., McLeod, A.Y., & Bunik, M. (2013). ABM Clinical Protocol #5: Peripartum breastfeeding management for the healthy mother and infant at term. *Breastfeeding Medicine, 8*(6), 469-473. Retrieved from https://www.bfmed.org/protocols.

45. Burke-Aaronson, A.C. (2015). Skin-to-skin care and breastfeeding in the perioperative suite. *American Journal of Maternal Child Nursing, 40*(2), 105-109.

46. Crenshaw, J.T. (2014). Healthy birth practice #6: Keep mother and baby together-It's best for mother, baby, and breastfeeding. *Journal of Perinatal Education, 23*(4), 211-217.

47. UNICEF UK Baby Friendly Initiative. (2017). *Guide to the UNICEF-UK Baby-Friendly Initiative standards* (2nd Ed.). London: UNICEF.

48. Widström, A. M., Lilja, G., Aaltomaa-Michalias, P., Dahllof, A., Lintula, M., & Nissen, E. (2011). Newborn behaviour to locate the breast when skin-to-skin: A possible method for enabling early self-regulation. *Acta Paediatrica Scandinavica, 100*, 79–85.

49. Flaherman, V.J., Hicks, K.G., Cabana, M.D., & Lee, K.A. (2012b). Maternal experience of interactions with providers among mothers with milk supply concern. *Clinical Pediatrics, 51*(8), 778–784.

50. Bystrova, K., Matthiesen A.S., Widstrom, A.M., Ransjo-Arvidson, A.B., Welles-Nystrom, B., Vorontsov, I., et al. (2007). The effect of Russian maternity home routines on breastfeeding and neonatal weight loss with special reference to swaddling. *Early Human Development, 83*, 29-39.

51. Colson, S., DeRooy, L., & Hawdon, J. (2003). Biological nurturing increases breastfeeding duration. *MIDIRS Midwifery Digest, 13*(1), 92-97.

52. Colson, S. (2006). *The mechanisms of biological nurturing.* PhD dissertation, Canterbury Christ Church University, Canterbury, UK.

53. Alberts, J.R. (1994). Learning as adaptation of the infant. *Acta Paediatrica,* 397(supplement), 77–85.

54. Colson, S., DeRooy, L., & Hawdon, J. (2003). Biological nurturing increases breastfeeding duration. *MIDIRS Midwifery Digest, 13*(1), 92-97.

55. Colson, S. (2008). Bringing nature to the fore. *Practising Midwife, 11*(10), 14-16, 18-19.

56. Hartmann, P.E. (1987). Lactation and reproduction in Western Australian women. *Reproductive Medicine, 32*, 543-547.
57. Hytten, F. (1995). *The clinical physiology of the puerperium.* London: Perrand Press.
58. Howie, P.W., Houston, M.J., Cook, A., Smart, L., McArdle, T., & McNeilly, A.S. (1981). How long should a breast-feed last? *Early Human Development, 5*, 71-77.
59. Brown, M.S., & Hurlock, J. T. (1975). Preparation of the breast for breastfeeding. *Nursing Research, 24*(6), 448-451.
60. Hytten, F. (1995). *The clinical physiology of the puerperium.* London: Perrand Press
61. Reader, F. (1996). The hospital experience. In K. Moss (Ed.). *Hidden loss* (2nd Ed.). London: The Women's Press.
62. McNeilly, A.S., Robinson, I.C.A., Houston, M.J., & Howie, P.W. (1983). Release of oxytocin and prolactin in response to suckling. *British Medical Journal, 286*, 257-259.
63. Howie, P.W. (1985). Breastfeeding: A new understanding. *Midwives, Chronicle and Nursing Notes, 7*, 184-192.
64. Uvnäs Moberg, K. (2003). *The oxytocin factor.* Cambridge, MA: Da Capo Press.
65. Morton, J. (2017). *Early hand expression increases later milk production.* Retrieved from https://med.stanford.edu/newborns/professional-education/breastfeeding/hand-expressing-milk.html.
66. Walker, M. (2014). *Breastfeeding management for the clinician: Using the evidence* (3rd Ed.). Sudbury, MA: Jones and Bartlett Publishers.
67. Hartmann, P.E., & Prosser, C.G. (1984). Physiological basis of longitudinal changes in human milk yield and composition. *Federation Proceedings, 43*, 2448-2453.
68. Bolling K., Grant, C., Hamlyn, B., & Thornton, K. (2007). *Infant feeding survey 2005.* London: The Information Centre.
69. Foster K., Lader, D., & Cheesbrough S. (1997). *Infant feeding 1995.* Office for National Statistics. London: The Stationery Office.
70. Hamlyn, B., Brooker, S., Oleinikova, K., & Wands S. (2002). *Infant feeding 2000.* London: TSO.
71. Martin, J., & Monk, J. (1982). *Infant feeding 1980.* Office of Population Censuses and Surveys. London: Social Survey Division, HMSO.
72. Martin, J., & White, A. (1987). *Infant feeding 1985.* Office of population Censuses and Surveys. London: Social Survey Division, HMSO.
73. McAndrew, F., Thompson, J., Fellows, L., Large, A., Speed, M., & Renfrew, M.J. (2012). *Infant Feeding Survey 2010.* Health and Social Care Information Centre. Retrieved from http://www.ic.nhs.uk/ statistics-and-data-collections/health-and-lifestyles-related-surveys/infant-feeding-survey/infant-feeding-survey-2010.
74. White, A., Freeth, S., & O'Brien, M. (1992). *Infant feeding 1990.* London: OPCS Social Survey Division HMSO.
75. Flaherman, V.J., Hicks, K.G., Cabana, M.D., & Lee, K.A. (2012b). Maternal experience of interactions with providers among mothers with milk supply concern. *Clinical Pediatrics, 51*(8), 778–784.
76. ibid
77. Stuebe, A.M., Grewen, K., & Meltzer-Brody, S. (2013). Association between maternal mood and oxytocin response to breastfeeding. *Journal of Women's Health, 22*(4), 352-361.
78. ibid
79. Pilliot, M. (2005). *Le regard du naissant. Cahiers de Maternologie, 23-24*, 65-80.
80. Woolridge, M.W., & Drewett, R. (1986). Sucking rates of human babies on the breast; a study using direct observation and intraoral pressure measurements. *Journal of Reproductive and Infant Psychology, 4*(1-2), 69-75.

CHAPTER 7: EXPLORATORY AND DESCRIPTIVE RESEARCH

1. Colson, S., DeRooy, L., & Hawdon, J. (2003). Biological nurturing increases breastfeeding duration. *MIDIRS Midwifery Digest, 13*(1), 92-97.
2. Quandt, S.A. (1998). Ecology of breastfeeding in the United States:

An applied perspective. *American Journal of Human Biology, 10*(2), 221-228.

3. Righard, L., & Alade, M.O. (1990). Effects of delivery room routines on success of first feed. *The Lancet, 336,* 1105-1107.

4. National Childbirth Trust. (1997). Hypoglycaemia of the newborn: New guidelines now available. *New Generation Digest, 19*(9). London: National Childbirth Trust.

5. De Rooy, L., & Hawdon, J.M. (2002). Nutritional factors that affect the postnatal metabolic adaptation of full-term small and large for gestational age infants. *Pediatrics, 109,* 42. Retrieved from http://pediatrics.aappublications.org/cgi/content/full/109/3/e42.

6. Colson, S. (2000). *Biological suckling facilitates exclusive breastfeeding from birth a pilot study of twelve vulnerable infants.* Unpublished master's dissertation. London: South Bank University.

7. Colson, S., DeRooy, L., & Hawdon, J. (2003). Biological nurturing increases breastfeeding duration. *MIDIRS Midwifery Digest, 13*(1), 92-97.

8. Medical Research Council (MRC) (2006) *Framework for the development and evaluation of complex interventions* retrieved 24 April 2019 from https://mrc.ukri.org/documents/pdf/complex-interventions-guidance/

9. Amiel-Tison, C., & Grenier, A. (1984). *La Surveillance Neurologique au cours de la Première Année de la Vie.* Paris: Masson.

10. André-Thomas, J.M., Chesni, Y., & Saint-Anne Dargassies, S. (1960). *The neurological examination of the infant.* London: The Medical Advisory Committee of the National Spastic Society.

11. Brazelton, T.B. & Nugent, J.K. (1995) *Neonatal Behavioural Assessment Scale* (3rd ed) London Mac Keith Press.

12. Dubowitz, L., Dubowitz, V., & Mercuri E. (1999). The neurological assessment of the preterm and the full-term newborn infant. *Clinics in developmental medicine.* Philadelphia: JB Lippincott.

13. Prechtl, H. (1977). *The neurological examination of the full term new born infant* (2nd Ed.). Clinics in Developmental Medicine, No 63. London: William Heinemann Books Ltd (Spastic International Medical Publications).

14. Colson, S.D., Meek J.H., & Hawdon, J.M. (2008). Optimal positions for the release of primitive neonatal reflexes stimulating breastfeeding. *Early Human Development, 84,* 441-449.

15. Anderson, G.C. (1989). Skin-to-skin: Kangaroo care in Western Europe. *American Journal of Nursing, 89,* 662-666.

16. Ludington-Hoe, S.M., with Golant, S.K. (1993). *Kangaroo care.* New York: Bantam Books.

17. Moore, E.R., Bergman, N., Anderson, G.C., & Medley, N. (2016). *Early skin-to-skin contact for mothers and their healthy newborn infants.* Cochrane Database of Systematic Reviews, 11. Retrieved from www.cochranelibrary.com

18. ibid

19. Roberts, K.L., Paynter, C., & McEwan, B. (2000). A comparison of kangaroo mother care and conventional cuddling care. *Neonatal Network, 19*(4), 31-35.

20. Anderson, G.C., Chiu, S-H., Dombrowski, M.A., Swinth, J.Y., Albert, J.M., & Wada, N. (2003). Mother-newborn contact in a randomized trial of kangaroo (skin-to-skin) care. *JOGNN, 32*(5), 604-611.

21. Hake-Brooks, S.J., & Anderson, G.C. (2008). Kangaroo care and breastfeeding of mother-preterm infant dyads 0-18 months: A randomized, controlled trial. *Neonatal Network, 27*(3), 151–159.

22. (Klaus & Kennel, 1976)

23. Hake-Brooks, S.J., & Anderson, G.C. (2008). Kangaroo care and breastfeeding of mother-preterm infant dyads 0-18 months: A randomized, controlled trial. *Neonatal Network, 27*(3), 151–159.

24. Colson, S. (2000). *Biological suckling facilitates exclusive breastfeeding from birth a pilot study of twelve vulnerable infants.* Unpublished master's dissertation. London: South Bank University.

25. Gadroy, D. (2016). *Naturellement votre. Mémoire de diplôme universitaire*

en lactation humaine et allaitement materne (DIULHAM). Retrieved from http://www.societe-francaise-neonatalogie.fr/2016/07/04/diu-lactation-humaine-allaitement-maternel-diulham/

CHAPTER 8: BIOLOGICAL NURTURING: THE ACTIVE INGREDIENTS AND MECHANISMS

1. Widström, A. M., Lilja, G., Aaltomaa-Michalias, P., Dahllof, A., Lintula, M., & Nissen, E. (2011). Newborn behaviour to locate the breast when skin-to-skin: A possible method for enabling early self-regulation. *Acta Paediatrica Scandinavica, 100,* 79–85.

CHAPTER 9: PRIMITIVE NEONATAL REFLEXES

1. Darwin, C. (1872). Biographical sketch of a small child. In A. Peiper (Ed.) (1963). *Cerebral function in infancy and childhood* (p. 417). New York: Consultants Bureau.
2. Preyer, W., (1893) *The mind of a child, Part I: The senses and the will.* (N.W. Brown, Trans.) New York: Appleton. Cited in Rosenblith, J.F. and Sims-Knight J.E., (1985) *In the Beginning Development in the first two years.* Monterey CA: Brooks/Cole Publishing Company,1-17
3. Peiper, A. (1963). *Cerebral function in infancy and childhood* (3rd Ed.) B. Nagler & H. Nagler (Trans.). New York: Consultants Bureau.
4. Piaget, J., (1955) *The Child's Construction of Reality.* London: Routledge and Kegan Paul Ltd
5. Illingworth, (1963) *The Development of the Infant and Young Child Normal and Abnormal.* (2nd Edition) Edinburgh: E. & S. Livingstone LTD
6. Gesell, A., Ilg, F.L. and Ames, L.B (1974) *Infant and Child in the Culture of Today.* London: Hamish Hamilton
7. Amiel-Tison, C., & Grenier, A. (1984). *La Surveillance Neurologique au cours de la Première Année de la Vie.* Paris: Masson.
8. André-Thomas, J.M., Chesni, Y., & Saint-Anne Dargassies, S. (1960). *The neurological examination of the infant.* London: The Medical Advisory Committee of the National Spastic Society.
9. Brazelton, T.B., & Nugent, K. (2011). *Neonatal Behavioural Assessment Scale* (4th Ed.). London: MacKeith Press.
10. Dubowitz, L., Dubowitz, V., & Mercuri E. (1999). The neurological assessment of the preterm and the full-term newborn infant. *Clinics in developmental medicine.* Philadelphia: JB Lippincott.
11. Prechtl, H. (1977). *The neurological examination of the full term new born infant* (2nd Ed.). Clinics in Developmental Medicine, No 63. London: William Heinemann Books Ltd (Spastic International Medical Publications).
12. Brazelton, T.B., & Nugent, K. (2011). *Neonatal Behavioural Assessment Scale* (4th Ed.). London: MacKeith Press.
13. Righard, L., & Frantz, K. (1992). *Delivery self attachment* [video]. Sunland, CA: Geddes Productions.
14. Widstrom, A.M., Ransjo-Arvidson, A.B., Matthiesen, A.S., Winberg, J., & Uvnäs Moberg, K. (1987). Gastric suction in healthy newborn infants. *Acta Paediatrica Scandanavica, 76,* 566-572.
15. Widstrom, A.M. (1996). *Breastfeeding: Baby's choice* [Videocassette]. Stockholm: Liber Utbildning.
16. Widström, A. M., Lilja, G., Aaltomaa-Michalias, P., Dahllof, A., Lintula, M., & Nissen, E. (2011). Newborn behaviour to locate the breast when skin-to-skin: A possible method for enabling early self-regulation. *Acta Paediatrica Scandinavica, 100,* 79–85.
17. Widström, A. M. (2013). *Breast crawl: Initiation of breastfeeding by breast crawl a scientific overview.* Retrieved from http://www.breastcrawl.org/science.shtml
18. Als, H. (1995). Manual for the naturalistic observation of newborn behaviour. *Newborn Individualized Developmental Care and Assessment Program* (NIDCAP). Boston: The Children's Hospital.
19. Nyqvist, K.H. (2005). Breastfeeding support in neonatal care: An example of the integration of international evidence and experience. *Newborn and Infant Nursing Reviews, 5*(1), 34–48.

20. Prechtl, H. (1977). *The neurological examination of the full term new born infant* (2nd Ed.). Clinics in Developmental Medicine, No 63. London: William Heinemann Books Ltd (Spastic International Medical Publications).
21. Amiel-Tison, C., & Grenier, A. (1984). *La Surveillance Neurologique au cours de la Première Année de la Vie.* Paris: Masson.
22. Dubowitz, L., Dubowitz, V., & Mercuri E. (1999). The neurological assessment of the preterm and the full-term newborn infant. *Clinics in developmental medicine.* Philadelphia: JB Lippincott.
23. Prechtl, H. (1977). *The neurological examination of the full term new born infant* (2nd Ed.). Clinics in Developmental Medicine, No 63. London: William Heinemann Books Ltd (Spastic International Medical Publications).
24. Brazelton, T.B., & Nugent, K. (2011). *Neonatal Behavioural Assessment Scale* (4th Ed.). London: MacKeith Press.
25. Prechtl, H.F. (2001). General movement assessment as a method of developmental neurology: New paradigms and their consequences. The 1999 Ronnie MacKeith lecture. *Developmental & Medical Child Neurology, 43*(12), 836-842.
26. Dubowitz, L., Dubowitz, V., & Mercuri, E. (1999). The neurological assessment of the preterm and the full-term newborn infant. *Clinics in developmental medicine.* Philadelphia: JB Lippincott.
27. Prechtl, H. (1977). *The neurological examination of the full term new born infant* (2nd Ed.). Clinics in Developmental Medicine, No 63. London: William Heinemann Books Ltd (Spastic International Medical Publications).
28. Colson, S.D., Meek J.H., & Hawdon, J.M. (2008). Optimal positions for the release of primitive neonatal reflexes stimulating breastfeeding. *Early Human Development, 84,* 441-449.
29. Bolling K., Grant, C., Hamlyn, B., & Thornton, K. (2007). *Infant feeding survey 2005.* London: The Information Centre.
30. Foster K., Lader, D., & Cheesbrough S. (1997). *Infant feeding 1995.* Office for National Statistics. London: The Stationery Office.
31. Hamlyn, B., Brooker, S., Oleinikova, K., & Wands S. (2002). *Infant feeding 2000.* London: TSO.
32. Martin, J., & Monk, J. (1982). *Infant feeding 1980.* Office of Population Censuses and Surveys. London: Social Survey Division, HMSO.
33. Martin, J., & White, A. (1987). *Infant feeding 1985.* Office of population Censuses and Surveys. London: Social Survey Division, HMSO.
34. McAndrew, F., Thompson, J., Fellows, L., Large, A., Speed, M., & Renfrew, M.J. (2012). *Infant Feeding Survey 2010.* Health and Social Care Information Centre. Retrieved from http://www.ic.nhs.uk/ statistics-and-data-collections/ health-and-lifestyles-related-surveys/infant-feeding-survey/infant-feeding-survey-2010.
35. White, A., Freeth, S., & O'Brien, M. (1992). *Infant feeding 1990.* London: OPCS Social Survey Division HMSO.
36. Gohil, J.R. (2006). Boxing neonate on an engorged breast: A new behaviour identified. *Journal of Human Lactation, 23*(3), 268–269.
37. ibid
38. World Health Organization (WHO). (1997). *Breast-feeding management: A modular course.* London: WHO/UNICEF, p. 94)
39. ibid
40. Peiper, A. (1963). *Cerebral function in infancy and childhood* (3rd Ed.) B. Nagler & H. Nagler (Trans.). New York: Consultants Bureau.
41. ibid
42. Hartmann, P.E. (1987). Lactation and reproduction in Western Australian women. *Reproductive Medicine, 32,* 543-547.
43. Brazelton, T.B., & Nugent, K. (2011). *Neonatal Behavioural Assessment Scale* (4th Ed.). London: MacKeith Press.
44. Hawdon, J.M., Ward-Platt, M.P., & Aynsley-Green, A. (1992). Patterns of metabolic

adaptation in term and preterm infants in the first postnatal week. *Archives of Diseases of Childhood, 67,* 357-365.

45. Riordan, J., & Hoover, K. (2010). Perinatal and intrapartum care. In J. Riordan & K. Wambach (Eds.), *Breastfeeding and human lactation* (4th Ed.). Boston, MA: Jones & Bartlett.

CHAPTER 10: MOTHER'S BREASTFEEDING POSTURES

1. Renfrew, M., Woolridge, M.W., & McGill, H.R. (2000). *Enabling breastfeeding.* London: TSO.
2. Renfrew, M., Dyson, L., Wallace, L., D'Souza, L., McCormick, F., & Spiby, H. (2005). *The effectiveness of public health interventions to promote the duration of breastfeeding systematic review* (1st Ed.). London: National Institute for Health and Clinical Excellence (NICE).
3. Royal College of Midwives. (2002). *Successful breastfeeding,* 3rd Ed. London: Churchill Livingstone.
4. Inch, S. (2003). Confusion surrounding breastfeeding terms 'positioning' and 'attachment'. *BJM (letter), 11*(3), 148.
5. Kapandji, I.A. (1974). *The physiology of the joints.* Vol.3. *The trunk and the vertebral column* (2nd Ed.). Edinburgh: Churchill Livingstone.
6. ibid p. 56
7. Kapandji, I.A. (1974). *The physiology of the joints.* Vol.3. *The trunk and the vertebral column* (2nd Ed.). Edinburgh: Churchill Livingstone.
8. ibid p. 112
9. ibid p. 112
10. Colson, S.D., Meek J.H., & Hawdon, J.M. (2008). Optimal positions for the release of primitive neonatal reflexes stimulating breastfeeding. *Early Human Development, 84,* 441-449.
11. Righard, L., & Frantz, K. (1992). *Delivery self attachment* [video]. Sunland, CA: Geddes Productions.
12. Sulcova, E. (1997). *Prague Newborn Behaviour Description Technique*: *Manual.* Prague: Psychiatric Centre, Laboratory of Psychometric Studies.
13. Righard, L., & Frantz, K. (1992). *Delivery self attachment* [video]. Sunland, CA: Geddes Productions.
14. Morris, D. (1977). *Manwatching: A field guide to human behaviour.* London: Triad/Panther Ltd.

CHAPTER 11: BABY'S BREASTFEEDING POSITIONS

1. Baston, H. (2014). Antenatal care. In J.E. Marshall & M.D. Raynor (Eds.), *Myles textbook for midwives,* 16th Ed. London: Churchill Livingstone Elsevier.
2. Cockburn, K.G., & Drake, R.F. (1969). Transverse and oblique lie of the foetus. *Obstetrical & Gynecological Survey, 24*(10), 1253-1255.
3. Wood, E.C., & Forster, F.M. (2005). Oblique and transverse foetal lie. *Obstetric and Gynecological Clinics of North America, 32*(2), 165-179.
4. McAndrew, F., Thompson, J., Fellows, L., Large, A., Speed, M., & Renfrew, M.J. (2012). *Infant Feeding Survey 2010.* Health and Social Care Information Centre. Retrieved from http://www.ic.nhs.uk/ statistics-and-data-collections/health-and-lifestyles-related-surveys/infant-feeding-survey/infant-feeding-survey-2010.
5. Baston, H. (2014). Antenatal care. In J.E. Marshall & M.D. Raynor (Eds.), *Myles textbook for midwives,* 16th Ed. London: Churchill Livingstone Elsevier.
6. Alberts, J.R., & Cramer C.P. (1988). Ecology and experience. In E.M. Blass (Ed.), *Developmental psychobiology and behavioural ecology. Handbook of behavioural neurobiology, Vol 9.* Boston, MA: Springer.
7. Woolridge, M.W., & Drewett, R. (1986). Sucking rates of human babies on the breast; a study using direct observation and intraoral pressure measurements. *Journal of Reproductive and Infant Psychology, 4*(1-2), 69-75.

8. Dubowitz, L., Dubowitz, V., & Mercuri E. (1999). The neurological assessment of the preterm and the full-term newborn infant. *Clinics in developmental medicine.* Philadelphia: JB Lippincott.

CHAPTER 12: LESSONS FROM OTHER MAMMALS

1. Stern, J. (2003). *Essentials of gross anatomy.* New York: F. A. Davis & Co.
2. Alberts, J.R. (1994). Learning as adaptation of the infant. *Acta Paediatrica,* 397(supplement), 77–85.
3. Stern, J. (2003). *Essentials of gross anatomy.* New York: F. A. Davis & Co.

CHAPTER 14: NEONATAL BEHAVIOURAL STATE

1. Brazelton T.B. (1961). Psychophysiologic reactions in the neonate, 1: The value of observation of the neonate. *Journal of Pediatrics, 58,* 508-512.
2. Brazelton, T.B., & Nugent, K. (2011). *Neonatal Behavioural Assessment Scale* (4th Ed.). London: MacKeith Press.
3. Blackburn, S.T. (2012). *Maternal, foetal, and neonatal physiology: A clinical perspective* (2nd Ed.). St Louis, MO: W.B. Saunders Company.
4. Brazelton, T.B., & Nugent, K. (2011). *Neonatal Behavioural Assessment Scale* (4th Ed.). London: MacKeith Press.
5. Mirmiran, M., Maas, Y.G.H., & Ariagno, R.L. (2003). Development of foetal and neonatal sleep and circadian rhythms. *Sleep Medicine Reviews, 7*(4), 321-334.
6. Blackburn, S.T. (2012). *Maternal, foetal, and neonatal physiology: A clinical perspective* (2nd Ed.). St Louis, MO: W.B. Saunders Company.
7. Brazelton, T.B., & Nugent, K. (2011). *Neonatal Behavioural Assessment Scale* (4th Ed.). London: MacKeith Press.
8. Nijhuis, J.G., Prechtl, H.F., Martin, C.B., Jr., & Bots, R.S. (1982). Are there behavioural states in the human foetus? *Early Human Development, 6,* 177-195.
9. Blackburn, S.T. (2012). *Maternal, foetal, and neonatal physiology: A clinical perspective* (2nd Ed.). St Louis, MO: W.B. Saunders Company.
10. Brazelton, T.B., & Nugent, K. (2011). *Neonatal Behavioural Assessment Scale* (4th Ed.). London: MacKeith Press.
11. Wolff, P.H. (1959). Observations on newborn infants. *Psychosomatic Medicine, 21,* 110-118.
12. Barnard, K., (2003). *NCAST-AVENUW Keys to Caregiving Program, Teaching Modules. Neonatal Behavioural State.* Seattle, WA: University of Washington.
13. ibid
14. Biancuzzo, M. (1999). *Breastfeeding the newborn. Clinical strategies for nurses.* St Louis, MO: Mosby.
15. Blackburn, S.T. (2012). *Maternal, foetal, and neonatal physiology: A clinical perspective* (2nd Ed.). St Louis, MO: W.B. Saunders Company.
16. Brazelton, T.B., & Nugent, K. (2011). *Neonatal Behavioural Assessment Scale* (4th Ed.). London: MacKeith Press.
17. Inch, S. (2014). Infant feeding. In J.E. Marshall & M.D. Raynor (Eds.), *Myles textbook for midwives,* 16th Ed. London: Churchill Livingstone Elsevier.
18. Koehn, M., & Riordan, J. (2010). Infant assessment. In J. Riordan & K. Wambach (Eds.), *Breastfeeding and human lactation* (4th Ed.). Boston, MA: Jones & Bartlett.
19. Prechtl, H. (1977). *The neurological examination of the full term new born infant* (2nd Ed.). Clinics in Developmental Medicine, No 63. London: William Heinemann Books Ltd (Spastic International Medical Publications).
20. UNICEF UK Baby Friendly Initiative UK. (2018). *Positioning and attachment* (Video). Retrieved from www.unicef-org.uk/BabyFriendly/Resources/AudioVideo/ Positioning-and-attachment.
21. Brazelton, T.B., & Nugent, K. (2011). *Neonatal Behavioural Assessment Scale* (4th Ed.). London: MacKeith Press.
22. ibid
23. Prechtl, H. (1977). *The neurological examination of the full term new born infant* (2nd Ed.).

Clinics in Developmental Medicine, No 63. London: William Heinemann Books Ltd (Spastic International Medical Publications).

24. UNICEF UK Baby Friendly Initiative UK. (2018). Co-sleeping* and SIDS: A guide for health professionals. Retrieved from https://www.unicef.org.uk/babyfriendly/wp-content/uploads/sites/2/2016/07/Co-sleeping-and- SIDS-A-Guide-for-Health-Professionals.pdf.

25. UNICEF UK Baby Friendly Initiative UK. (2018). Caring for your baby at night. Retrieved from https://www.unicef.org.uk/babyfriendly/ baby-friendly-resources/sleep-and-night-time-resources/ caring-for-your-baby-at-night/

26. Knowles, R. (2016). *Why babywearing matters.* London: Pinter & Martin.

27. Montagu, A. (1971). *Touching: The human significance of the skin.* New York: Harper & Row Publishers.

CHAPTER 15: MATERNAL HORMONAL STATE

1. Uvnäs Moberg, K. (2003). *The oxytocin factor.* Cambridge, MA: Da Capo Press.
2. ibid
3. Herbert, J. (1994). Oxytocin and sexual behaviour. *British Medical Journal, 309,* 891-892.
4. Pedersen, C.A. (1992). Oxytocin in maternal sexual and social behaviours. *Annals of the New York Academy of Sciences,* 652, IX-XI.
5. Uvnäs Moberg, K. (2013). *The hormone of closeness: The role of oxytocin in relationships.* London: Pinter & Martin.
6. ibid
7. Uvnäs Moberg, K. (1989). Physiological and psychological effects of oxytocin and prolactin in connection with motherhood with special reference to food intake and the endocrine system of the gut. *Acta Physiologica Scandinavica, 136 Supplementum, 583,* 41-48.
8. Nissen, E., Uvnäs Moberg, K., Svensson, K., Stock, S., Widstrom, A.M., & Winberg, J. (1996). Different patterns of oxytocin, prolactin but not cortisol release during breastfeeding in women delivered by Caesarean section or by the vaginal route. *Early Human Development, 45,* 103-118.
9. Uvnäs Moberg, K. (1997). Oxytocin linked anti-stress effects–the relaxation and growth response. *Acta Physiologica Scandinavia Supplementum, 584,* 38-42.
10. Uvnäs Moberg, K. (1998). Anti-stress pattern induced by oxytocin. *News in Physiological Science, 13,* 22-26.
11. Pedersen, C.A. (1992). Oxytocin in maternal sexual and social behaviours. *Annals of the New York Academy of Sciences,* 652, IX-XI.
12. Walker, M. (2014). *Breastfeeding management for the clinician: Using the evidence* (3rd Ed.). Sudbury, MA: Jones and Bartlett Publishers.
13. Bentley, G.R. (1998). Hydration as a limiting factor in lactation. *American Journal of Human Biology, 10,* 151-161.
14. Colson, S., & Greenfield, T. (2006). Maternal hormonal complexion, a theory. In S. Colson (Ed.), *The mechanisms of biological nurturing.* Doctoral thesis, Canterbury Christ Church University, Canterbury, UK.

CHAPTER 16: INSTINCTUAL BREASTFEEDING

1. Rothman, B.K. (1985). *In Labour: Women and power in the birthplace.* London: Junction books Ltd.
2. Roper, N., Logan, W.W., & Tierney, A.J. (2000). *The Roper, Logan, and Tierney model of nursing based on activities of living* (4th Ed.). London: Churchill Livingstone.
3. (Colson et al., 2008, p. 446)
4. ibid
5. McFarland, D. (2006). *A dictionary of animal behaviour.* Oxford, UK: Oxford University Press.

APPENDIX:
BIOLOGICAL NURTURING RESEARCH

Brief Summary

The so called biological nurturing (BN) – or laid-back breastfeeding (LB BF), a new neurobehavioural approach to breastfeeding (BF), has the potential to enhance BF initiation and to reduce breast problems (pain, fissures, etc.), while easing the newborn attachment to the breast. BN focuses on facilitating the mother to breastfeed in a relaxed, laid-back position, with her baby laying prone on her, so that the baby's body is in the largest possible contact with mother's curves. This position opens up the mother's body and promotes baby's movements through the activation of 20 primary neonatal reflexes stimulating BF. Neurophysiological studies show that, through this approach, infants instinctively know how to feed, thanks to the presence of neonatal reflexes, at the same time mothers being able to instinctively activate the same reflexes.

The main objective of this study is to assess the effectiveness of LB BF compared to standard hospital practices on the frequency of breast problems (i.e., pain, fissures, etc.) at discharge.

For more information go to https://bit.ly/2EeigzO and scroll down to clinical trial laid-back breastfeeding.

ABOUT THE AUTHOR

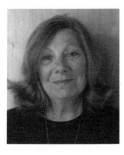

Dr. Suzanne Colson is a midwife and a nurse. Her thesis introduced a new breastfeeding paradigm called biological nurturing and won the prestigious English Royal College of Nursing Inaugural Akinsanya Award for originality and scholarship in doctoral studies. Suzanne is an Ankinsanya scholar 2007 and a visiting principal research fellow at Canterbury Christ Church University. She is an honorary member and a founding mother/leader of La Leche League France. She is also on the professional advisory board of La Leche League of Great Britain.

Suzanne has more than 40 years clinical experience supporting breastfeeding mothers in both hospital and community settings. She worked in Pithiviers, France as a lactation consultant with Dr. Michel Odent and as a caseload midwife and a baby feeding advisor in the NHS. Passionate about research, she worked on the Williams, Hawdon and DeRooy team examining the effects of supplementation on metabolic adaptation and breastfeeding and studied a subset of mother-baby pairs for her MSc.

Suzanne is the author of numerous articles, research papers, a book, translated into 4 languages and three DVDs. Retired from active midwifery practice, she has been interviewed on BBC radio, appeared on breakfast TV and presented the biological nurturing research in 21 countries across the world. She currently organises 5-day biological nurturing certification workshops and remains available for clinical consultation.

INDEX

A

agitated states 136–7, 139, 143
Alberts, J.R. 32, 33, 46, 122, 128
analgesia 21
angle of approach to breast, baby's 13, 82, 97, 118
antenatal education 3, 56, 57
anxiety 51, 58, 61–2, 148, 152, 163
archaic reflexes see primitive neonatal reflexes (PNRs)
arched-back nursing 128
arm cycling see cycling movements
arms, mother's (freedom of) 27, 97, 111, 126
artificial milk drink (formula) 19, 50, 55, 56, 100
attitude, baby's 26–7, 78, 82, 119–24, 126
awake states 136–7

B

Babinski toe fan reflex 43, 86, 88, 99, 126
Baby Friendly Initiative (BFI) 30, 46, 51, 52, 89
babywearing 145
back, baby's (no need for supporting) 27, 82, 91, 95, 132–3
back, supported (mother) 6, 80–1, 111, 148
Barnard, Kathryn 137
bedsharing guidelines 144–5
behaving body 33, 46–8, 50, 54, 59, 122
behavioural states 78, 135–46, 147–54
blood sugar 23, 34, 49, 58, 100, 162
body nest, mothers make a 27, 44, 127, 141, 156
body placing 157
bonding 57, 58, 82, 162
bony pelvis 102–5
bottle feeding 16–17, 19, 54, 100
brain development 28, 100
brain plasticity 59
Brazelton, T.B. 28, 29, 84, 135, 136, 137, 141
breast boxing 89, 139
breast crawl 37, 43, 71, 85, 109
breast emptying 53, 60, 63, 100
breast refusal 89, 139
breasts, sexualisation of 16
brushing 6, 28–9, 85, 100, 118, 132, 139

C

Cadogan, William 10–11
caesarean births 107, 111, 121
cardinal reflex 89, 122, 123, 140
cheek-to-breast sleeping 2, 8, 30, 34, 39, 74, 122, 142
chin-leading 13, 15, 62, 122–3
colostrum 50, 51–2, 54–5, 58, 60, 63
comfortable posture, encouraging mother to choose 6, 131
comforting/calming baby, breastfeeding for 51
'coming in,' milk 59–60
compression of breast 44
conditioning reflexes 58, 99, 100, 110, 113, 141–2
continuity 25–32, 116, 150–1, 162
co-sleeping 144–5
cots 31, 35, 51, 56, 60, 62–3, 138, 141, 145
counterregulation 49, 55, 56
cradle hold 93, 116, 118
crawling reflex 20, 22, 85, 88
critical periods 57–9
cross-cradle hold 93, 116, 118
crying 46, 61, 63, 82, 135, 138–40, 143, 145
cup feeding 51, 54, 56
curve of spine 127–9
cycling movements 28, 88, 89, 91, 140

D

dance, mother-baby 6
decoy feeding 54
deep sleep states 29, 61, 135, 136, 138, 140, 141, 142, 145
demand feeding 22, 51–2, 60
Deshpande, S. 49–50
diabetes 23
discontinuity 56–64, 162

dorsal feeding 91, 97, 107, 126, 130–1
see also upright positions
dress state 48, 71–2, 113 *see also* skin-to-skin
drowsy states 136–7, 138, 140, 142
Dubowitz model 85–6
duration of breastfeeding 30–2, 53, 61, 68, 69, 71–5

E

en face gaze 73
endogenous drives 55, 88, 98–9
engorgement 58, 89, 145
Entwistle, F. 16, 52
erect nipples 151, 152
estrogen 60
exhaustion, newborn 46
expert, mother as 78, 155–60
expression of milk 51–5, 59, 162

F

facial reflexes 122–3
feeding cues
baby 22, 51, 63, 137, 139–40
maternal 22, 74
feeding frenzy 60
feeding records 19–20, 65–6
feet, supported (baby's) 27, 43, 91, 94, 95, 121
fighting the breast 56, 58, 88, 89, 145
finger extension/flexion 140
finger feeding 54
finger grasping reflex 86, 88
finger sucking 22, 51, 89
first 24 hours 51–4, 67–8
first hour after birth 20, 51, 57–9
flat-lying positions 105
flexion/extension degree 62, 86, 119–24, 126
foetal behavioural states 136
foetal lie and attitude, continuity with 26, 62, 115, 116
foetal movement 27
foot reflexes 43, 99 *see also specific reflexes*
forward movement, baby's 43
Frantz, Kittie 20
frequency of feeding 50, 54, 100, 137–8
frontal feeding 91–5, 97

G

gape 91, 98, 140
Gaskin, Ina May 134
gaze/eye-contact 6, 63, 73, 80, 82, 148, 152, 156, 158
gestational age 84, 86, 124
Glabella 122–3
glucose 23, 34, 49, 55, 100, 162
glycogen reserves 49, 56
golden hour 20, 51, 57–9
good fit 27, 121–4, 125
gravity
anti-gravity reflexes 88
frontal feeding 95
mechanisms of biological nurturing 5–6, 80, 82, 83, 131, 132–4
and the rooting reflex 90
guilt 61, 99
Gunther, Mavis 12–13

H

habitat 33, 38, 50, 59, 62, 122, 129 *see also* right address, baby at the
hand expression 51–5, 58, 59, 162–3
hand/finger sucking 22, 51, 89
hands-on support 44–5
hand-to-mouth reflex 85, 89, 90, 140
Hawdon, Jane 23, 49–50, 65
Hawthorne effect 73
head bobbing 62, 78, 88, 91, 98, 116, 122, 140
health professionals
latching baby on 44–5
in modern methods of breastfeeding 9, 13, 155
mother's dependence on 155–7
and oxytocin 151, 154
role is to manage environment 5, 26, 78, 158, 163
holding babies for prolonged periods 22, 23, 66–8, 73–4, 82, 144–5, 161–2
hormonal complexion 151–3
hormonal state, mother's 4–5, 31–2, 150–3
hospital births 12–13, 50
hunger and interest 98–100
hyperextension 122, 124, 126
hypoglycaemia 23, 34, 55, 65

I

imprinting behaviours 54, 141, 163
Inch, Sally 13, 28, 102
indeterminate sleep states 29–30, 99, 136, 141, 142
initiation of breastfeeding 22, 37, 66, 70, 72, 75, 85, 100, 140–5
instinctual behaviour, breastfeeding as 9–17, 148, 155–60
insufficient milk, perceptions of 59–60, 61, 63, 144
interest in breastfeeding 99–100
invitations to feed 22

J

jerky movements 28, 42–3, 88, 132, 139

K

kangaroo care 22, 71, 72–3
ketone bodies 23, 49, 50, 55, 100
Kitzinger, Sheila 134
koala hold 126

L

La Leche League 18, 22
lactate bodies 49, 55
"laid-back breastfeeding" 4
laid-back sitting positions 79, 80, 82, 104–5
language of breastfeeding 15–16
latch
    and baby's facial reflexes 123
    and baby's lie position 117, 118
    in biological nurturing 80, 82, 120
    failure of 89–90
    and 'good fit' 121–2
    and gravity 110
    and hunger/interest in breastfeeding 99
    latch reflex 63
    link with foot reflexes 99
    mother guides 44, 157
    and mother's position 108–9
    no one single "correct" 62, 163
    not necessarily preceded by rooting 78
    and primitive newborn reflexes 88, 89–90
    self-attachment 37, 44, 46, 98, 109,

116
    and semi-reclined positions 108
    during sleep 137, 139
    symmetry of 123–4, 163
    techniques taught to midwives 13
    time taken to self-attach 44
    and upright positions 89–91
latchments 54
learned/acquired skill, breastfeeding seen as 157
learning body habitat 38, 55
learning to breastfeed 9–15
left-hand side 42
leg cycles see cycling movements
licking 78, 85, 140
lie, baby's 26–7, 78, 82, 98, 115–19
light sleep see drowsy states; indeterminate sleep states; REM sleep states
lip diamonds 122–3
lip smacking 22, 51, 140
lipogenesis 49
longitudinal lie 98, 116, 117, 118, 121
lordosis 128

M

Masseter (jaw jerk) reflex 88, 122–3
maternal comfort mechanisms 111–12
maternal continuity 31–2
medicalisation of infant feeding 10–11
metabolic adaptation 34, 48, 49–50, 61, 82, 141, 162
midwife education 13–15, 16–17, 162
milk supply and demand processes 53–4
milk transfer 13, 60–3, 66–7, 80, 88, 99, 108, 163
milk-ejection reflex 133
mimicry 11–12
Mobbs, Elsie 54
Moro reflex 84
Morris, Desmond 10, 42, 44, 113
Morton, Jane 51
mother/baby suckling diaries 22–3, 66, 68
mother-centred approach 4, 48, 155–63
mouthing 78
muscle tone 64, 85

N

nakedness, not necessary 7, 37, 72, 162
nappies 64
nature versus nurture 9–15
navel radiation 27, 28, 29, 139
Neonatal Behavioural Assessment Scale
  (NBAS) 28, 141
nervous system, baby's 28, 84–5, 135–6
nest, mothers make with body 27, 44,
  127, 141, 156
neurological assessment 85- 6
niche 33, 63, 129
nipple-to-nose 13

O

oblique lie 116, 117, 118
Odent, M. 134
oxytocin
  and anxiety 58, 61–2, 163
  and biological nurturing 4–5, 82
  hand expression versus active
    suckling 55
  health professionals' role in guarding
    158, 163
  and hospital birth 13
  and maternal continuity 31–2
  and maternal gaze 148
  and milk production 60
  and posture 5
  role of 149–51
  threats to 152

P

pain (mother's) 108, 111
palmar grasp reflex 88
Peiper, A. 84, 91, 94, 131
pelvis 102–5
pendular movements 94, 95
pethidine 21
placing reflex 43, 86, 87, 88, 121, 126
plantar grasp reflex 43, 86, 88, 99
poo 64
positional stability 91, 95, 121, 125,
  126, 129
positioning-and-attachment (P & A)
  skills 22
postnatal depression 61
posture, maternal 78, 79–81, 88, 91–5,
  101–14, 127
Prechtl, H.F.R. 28, 42, 85, 86, 94, 135

preterm babies 23, 29, 34, 59, 62, 66, 72
primates 12, 129, 130
primitive neonatal reflexes (PNRs) 29,
  82, 84–100, 108, 122, 137, 139, 140
privacy, protecting mothers' 16, 48,
  112–14, 163
prolactin 60, 158, 163
prone positions 27, 28, 42, 71, 86, 95,
  99, 122
protogaze 63, 162
Pryor, Karen 12
public, breastfeeding in 16, 112 14
public health approaches to
  breastfeeding 10, 162

Q

quadrupeds, human babies as 1, 82, 83,
  127–9
quiet alert states 30, 99, 137, 138, 143

R

rates of breastfeeding 23–4, 34, 35, 52,
  68, 162
reflex diamonds of a baby's face 122–3
reflexes *see also specific reflexes*
  and biological nurturing 68
  continuity in 29
  jerky movements 28, 42–3, 88, 132,
    139
  primitive neonatal reflexes (PNRs)
    29, 82, 84–100, 108, 122, 137, 139,
    140
  rhythmic reflexes 88, 123
  in the womb 24
relationship, breastfeeding as 4, 44, 83,
  155–60
REM sleep states 82, 135, 136, 137,
  138, 140, 141, 142
research design 69–71
responsive breastfeeding 51–2
responsive mothering 161
rhythmic reflexes 88, 123
right address, baby at the 7, 32, 33–48,
  50, 60, 63, 82, 122, 145, 162
rooming-in 35–7
rooting reflex 20, 22, 78, 85, 88, 89–90,
  116, 122, 140
rousing techniques 51
rugby/football hold 93, 116, 118

S

sacral sitting 78, 104, 107, 148, 153
scheduled feeding 11, 60
self-attachment 37, 44, 46, 98, 109, 116
self-soothing 161–2
semi-ischial sitting 78, 104, 107
semi-reclined positions 94–5, 101–14, 148 see also slope of mother's body
sensory awakening 63
separation of mother and baby 20–2, 25, 31, 35, 56, 162
"settled" after a feed 61, 62–3
side-lying positions 13, 91, 93, 97, 105, 108
side-to-side head movements 89
skin-to-skin 6–7, 16, 20, 37–8, 71–4, 85, 162
sleep
    after feeding 62–3
    at the breast 82, 99
    cheek-to-breast sleeping 2, 8, 30, 34, 39, 74, 122, 142
    feeding during 7, 30, 137, 140–4, 162
    during first 24 hours 51
    foetal 136
    neonatal behavioural states 135–46
sleep cycles 6, 29–31, 136, 141, 145
slings 145
slope of mother's body 43, 83, 94–5, 101–14, 127
small-for-gestational-age infants 23
sore nipples 6, 58, 82, 108, 111, 118, 133, 145
spinal anatomy 127–9
spoon feeding 51, 54, 56
stepping reflex 20, 84, 85, 88, 126
Stern, Jack 127
sucking reflex 85, 88
suckling ketosis 23
sudden infant death (SID) 27
sufficient milk, gauging 61–3
Sulcova, E. 109
swaddling 13, 28, 51
swallowing 55, 60, 63, 64, 67, 74, 85, 99
swallowing reflex 85, 88
syringe feeding 51

T

thirst, mother's 151, 152
transverse lie 91, 98, 116, 119, 120
trigeminal area of baby's face 62, 95, 98, 122
Truby King, Frederick 11
tummy pressure 6–7, 27, 28, 80
twins 124

U

upright positions
    compared to biological nurturing positions 97
    and foetal lie 116–18
    and gravity 132
    ischial sitting 102, 104, 107
    for labour and birth 134
    and latch failure 89–91
    morality of 130–1
    mother bipedal, neonate quadruped 129–31
    mother's behavioural state 147
    other mammals 125–6
    and primitive newborn reflexes 108
    as protection for mother's frontal region 113
    reasons for using 108–11
    taught to midwives 13
Uvnäs Moberg, Kerstin 149, 150, 151, 153

V

veiling 160
ventral contact positions 27, 80, 81, 82, 122, 139
ventral suspension 86–7, 157
vertical football hold 126
volume of milk taken 19, 59–60, 63
vomiting 19

W

Walker, Marsha 150–1
Ward Platt, M. 49–50
weight gain 56, 61–3
wet nappies 64
Widström, A.M. 37, 43, 46, 85
womb feeding 25, 27, 33, 48, 49, 50, 82, 162
woodpecker (head-bob) reflex see head bobbing
writhing 28